D1131780

Series Editor

Prof. Dr. Michael J. Parnham
PLIVA
Research Institute
Prilaz baruna Filipovica 25
10000 Zagreb
Croatia

Cytokines and Pain

Linda R. Watkins
Steven F. Maier

Editors

Birkhäuser Verlag
Basel · Boston · Berlin

Editors

Prof. Dr. Linda R. Watkins
Prof. Dr. Steven F. Maier
Dept. of Psychology
University of Colorado at Boulder
Boulder, CO 80309-0345
USA

A CIP catalogue record for this book is available from the Library of Congress, Washington D.C., USA

Deutsche Bibliothek Cataloging-in-Publication Data
Cytokines and pain / ed. by L.R. Watkins, S.F. Maier... - Basel ; Boston ;
Berlin : Birkhäuser, 1999
    (Progress in inflammation research)
    ISBN 3-7643-5849-1 (Basel...)
    ISBN 0-8176-5849-1 (Boston)

The publisher and editor can give no guarantee for the information on drug dosage and administration contained in this publication. The respective user must check its accuracy by consulting other sources of reference in each individual case.

The use of registered names, trademarks etc. in this publication, even if not identified as such, does not imply that they are exempt from the relevant protective laws and regulations or free for general use.

This work is subject to copyright. All rights are reserved, whether the whole or part of the material is concerned, specifically the rights of translation, reprinting, re-use of illustrations, recitation, broadcasting, reproduction on micro-films or in other ways, and storage in data banks. For any kind of use, permission of the copyright owner must be obtained.

© 1999 Birkhäuser Verlag, P.O. Box 133, CH-4010 Basel, Switzerland
Printed on acid-free paper produced from chlorine-free pulp. TCF ∞
Cover design: Markus Etterich, Basel
Cover illustration: With the friendly permission of Dr. Joyce A. DeLeo, Dartmouth-Hitchcock Medical Center, Lebanon, USA
Printed in Germany
ISBN 3-7643-5849-1
ISBN 0-8176-5849-1

Contents

List of contributors

Andrea L. Clatworthy, Department of Biology, University of North Carolina at Charlotte, 9201 University City Blvd., Charlotte, NC 28223, USA; e-mail: aclatwor@email.uncc.edu

Raymond W. Colburn, Dartmouth-Hitchcock Medical Center, Departments of Anesthesiology and Pharmacology, 1 Medical Center Drive, HB 7125, Lebanon, NH 03756, USA; e-mail: Raymond.W.Colburn@Dartmouth.edu

Fernando de Queiroz Cunha, Department of Pharmacology, Faculty of Medicine of Ribeirão Preto, University of São Paulo, Ribeirão Preto, Brazil; e-mail: fdqcunha@fmrp.usp.br

Joyce A. DeLeo, Dartmouth-Hitchcock Medical Center, Departments of Anesthesiology and Pharmacology, 1 Medical Center Drive, HB 7125, Lebanon, NH 03756, USA; e-mail: Joyce.A.DeLeo@Dartmouth.edu

Charles A. Dinarello, Department of Medicine, Division of Infectious Diseases, B168, University of Colorado Health Center, 4200 East Ninth Ave., Denver, CO 80262, USA

Sergio Henriques Ferreira, Department of Pharmacology, Faculty of Medicine of Ribeirão Preto, University of São Paulo, Ribeirão Preto, Brazil; e-mail: shferrei@fmrp.usp.br

Tetsuro Hori, Department of Physiology, Kyushu University, Faculty of Medicine, Fukuoka 812-8582 Japan; e-mail: thori@physiol.med.kyushu-u.ac.jp

Steven F. Maier, Department of Psychology, Campus Box 345, University of Colorado at Boulder, Boulder, CO 80309-0345, USA; e-mail: smaier@psych.colorado.edu

D. Martin, Department of Pharmacology, Amgen Inc., One Amgen Center Drive, Thousand Oaks, CA 91320, USA

Robert R. Myers, VA Medical Center and the University of California, San Diego (0629), Departments of Anesthesiology and Pathology, 9500 Gilman Drive, La Jolla, CA 92093-0629, USA; e-mail: rmyers@ucsd.edu

Takakazu Oka, Departments of Psychosomatic Medicine and Physiology, Kyushu University, Faculty of Medicine, Fukuoka 812-8582 Japan; e-mail: toka@cephal.med.kyushu-u.ac.jp

Stephen Poole, Division of Endocrinology, National Institute for Biological Standards and Control, Blanche Lane, South Mimms, Potters Bar, Herts EN6 3QG, UK; e-mail: spoole@nibsc.ac.uk

Linda S. Sorkin, VA Medical Center and the University of California, San Diego (0629), Department of Anesthesiology, 9500 Gilman Drive, La Jolla, CA 92093-0629, USA; e-mail: lsorkin@ucsd.edu

Rochelle Wagner, VA Medical Center and the University of California, San Diego (0629), Department of Anesthesiology, 9500 Gilman Drive, La Jolla, CA 92093-0629, USA

Linda R. Watkins, Department of Psychology, Campus Box 345, University of Colorado at Boulder, Boulder, CO 80309-0345, USA; e-mail: lwatkins@psych.colorado.edu

Clifford J. Woolf, Neural Plasticity Research Group, Dept. of Anesthesia, Massachusetts General Hospital and Harvard Medical School, 149 13th Street, Room 4309, Charlestown, MA 02129, USA

Overview of inflammatory cytokines and their role in pain

Charles A. Dinarello

Department of Medicine, Division of Infectious Diseases, University of Colorado Health Sciences Center, 4200 East Ninth Avenue, Denver, CO 80262, USA

Introduction

Cytokines are small, non-structural proteins with molecular weights ranging from 8–40,000 Daltons. Originally called lymphokines and monokines to indicate their cellular sources, it became clear that the term "cytokine" is the best description since nearly all nucleated cells are capable of synthesising of these proteins and, in turn, respond to them. There is no amino acid sequence motif or three dimensional structure that links cytokines; rather, their biological activities allow us to group them into different classes. For the most part, cytokines are primarily involved in host responses to disease or infection and any involvement with homeostatic mechanisms has been less than dramatic. At least that is the present wisdom derived from gene deletion studies in mice.

Many scientists have made the analogy of cytokines to hormones but upon closer examination, this is not an accurate comparison. Why? First, hormones tend to be constitutively expressed by highly specialized tissues but cytokines are synthesized by nearly every cell. Whereas hormones are the primary synthetic product of a cell (insulin, thyroid hormone, ACTH, etc.), cytokines account for a very small amount of the synthetic output of a cell. In addition, hormones are expressed in response to homeostatic control signals, many of which are part of a daily cycle. In contrast, most cytokine genes are not expressed (at least at the translational level) unless specifically stimulated by noxious events. In fact, it has become clear that the kinases involved in triggering cytokine gene expression are triggered by a variety of "cell stressors". For example, ultraviolet light, heat-shock, hyperosmolarity, or adherence to a foreign surface activate the mitogen-activated protein kinases (MAPK) which phosphorylate transcription factors for gene expression. Of course, infection and inflammatory products also use the MAPK pathway for initiating cytokine gene expression. One concludes then that cytokines themselves are produced in response to "stress" whereas most hormones are produced by a daily intrinsic clock.

Cytokines and Pain, edited by Linda R. Watkins and Steven F. Maier
© 1999 Birkhäuser Verlag Basel/Switzerland

Cytokine responses to infection

Based on their primary biological activities, cytokines are often grouped as lymphocyte growth factors, mesenchymal growth factors, interferons, chemokines, and colony-stimulating factors. Some have been given the name "interleukin" (IL) to indicate a product of a leukocyte and a target leukocyte cell. There are presently eighteen cytokines with the name "interleukin" (IL-1 through IL-18). The name "interleukin" is assigned to molecules with a biological activity associated with a novel human DNA sequence. The gene product is expressed in a recombinant form and shown to be the same as the natural product. Other cytokines have retained their original biological description such as "tumor necrosis factor" (TNF). Another way to look at some cytokines is their role in inflammation and this is particularly relevant to the importance of inflammation to pain. Hence, some cytokines clearly promote inflammation and are called pro-inflammatory cytokines, whereas others suppress the activity of pro-inflammatory cytokines and are called anti-inflammatory cytokines.

Cytokines tend to be rather promiscuous with respect to their choice of partners. For example, IL-4 and IL-10 are potent activators of B lymphocytes which are responsible for antibody formation to a foreign (or endogenous) antigen. Cytokines which "help" promote B cells antibody formation are classed as T lymphocyte helper cell of the type 2 class (Th2). The counterpart to T lymphocyte helper cells of the type 2 class are cytokines that "help" the type 1 T-lymphocytes (Th1). Th1 cytokines "help" the process of cellular immunity in which T-lymphocytes attack and kill virus-infected cells. Th1 cytokines include IL-2, IL-12, IL-18 and interferon-γ (IFNγ). However, IL-4 and IL-10, although both initially discovered for being Th2 cytokines, are also both potent anti-inflammatory agents. These are anti-inflammatory cytokines by virtue of their ability to suppress genes for pro-inflammatory cytokines such as IL-1, TNF, and the chemokines.

IFNγ is another example of the pleiotropic nature of cytokines. Although like IFNα and IFNβ, IFNγ possesses anti-viral activity and is also an activator of the Th1 response which leads to cytotoxic T cells. IFNγ is also considered a pro-inflammatory cytokine because it augments TNF activity and induces nitric oxide (NO). Therefore, listing cytokines in various categories should be done with an open mind in that, depending upon the biological process, any cytokine may function differentially. For example, in the brain, T-lymphocytes are rarely found unless there is an immunologically driven disease. IL-10 in the brain functions primarily to reduce the inflammation resulting from IL-1 production. Following blunt trauma to the brain there is bleeding and microglia produce IL-1. IL-1 then increases prostaglandin E_2 (PGE$_2$) production and contributes to brain swelling but the local production of IL-10 in the traumatized brain likely limits the production of IL-1 and hence limits the extent of inflammation. In this regard, mice deficient in IL-10 (mice with a null mutation for IL-10) will have an exaggerated inflammatory response to injury.

Table 1 - Classes of cytokines

Lymphocyte growth factors	IL-2; IL-4; IL-6; IL-7; IL-9; IL-10; IL-12; IL-13; IL-14; IFNγ
Colony stimulating factors	G-CSF, IL-3; GM-CSF; Erythropoietin, Thrombopoietin; M-CSF, IL-11
Chemokines	IL-8; MIP's, Rantes, etc. (There are over 20 genes coding for chemokines.)
Pro-inflammatory	IL-1; TNF; IL-17; IL-18; chemokines
Anti-inflammatory	IL-1Ra; IL-10; IL-4; TGFβ; LIF
Interferons	IFNα; IFNβ
Mesenchymal growth factors	TGFβ; FGF; PDGF; VEGF; NGF; CNTF; cardiotropin-1

Although this particular experiment has not been reported, when challenged with endotoxin, IL-10-deficient mice have more inflammation than the wild-type control mice. Table 1 lists some commonly studied cytokines arrayed into different classes.

Figure 1 illustrates some of the major cytokine pathways involved in orchestrating the T cell and immune responses to infection. It should be pointed out that these same cytokines (IFNγ, IL-6, IL-10, IL-4) are also major participants in directly controlling inflammation and hence serve as an example of the pleiotropic nature of cytokines.

The concept of pro- and anti-inflammatory cytokines and their relationship to pain

For the most part, pain is associated with inflammation. Nerve endings sense the swelling of local tissues which is a hallmark of inflammation, the other hallmark being erythema. The injection of pro-inflammatory cytokines locally into humans results in pain, swelling, and erythema. The concept that some cytokines function primarily to induce inflammation whereas others suppress inflammation is fundamental to cytokine biology and also to clinical medicine. The concept is based on the genes coding for small molecules that are upregulated during inflammation. For example, genes that are pro-inflammatory are phospholipase A_2 type-II, cyclooxygenase-2 (COX-2), and inducible nitric oxide synthase (iNOS). These genes code for enzymes which increase synthesis of platelet activating factor and leukotrienes, prostanoids and nitric oxide. Another class of genes that are pro-inflammatory are chemokines and endothelial adhesion molecules. Taken together, cytokine-mediated inflammation is a cascade of gene products usually not produced while in a healthy state. What triggers the expression of these genes? Although inflammatory products do so, the cytokines IL-1 and TNF are particularly effective in stimulating the

3

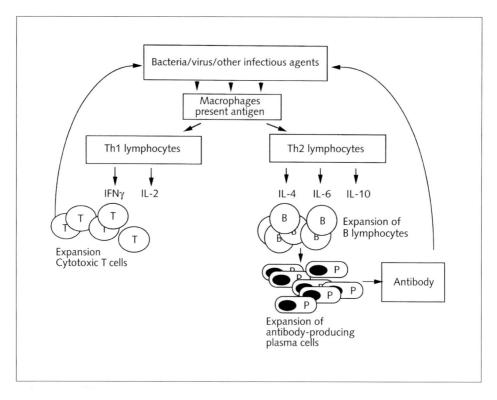

Figure 1
Cytokine pathways in the immune response to infection.
Infectious agents are foreign antigens and trigger immune responses which are designed to eliminate the invader either by cell-mediated (called Th1) or antibody-mediated (called Th2) mechanisms. The first encounter with the host macrophages results in the killing of the organisms but also present critical microbial antigens to T lymphocytes. The T-lymphocytes that "help" the pathways for TH1 responses produce IFNγ and IL-2. These cytokines are growth factors for Th1 cells and leads to clonal expansion of cytotoxic T cells which, in turn, attack the invading organism (usually viruses inside cells). Th2 cytokines such as IL-4, IL-6 and IL-10 stimulate expansion of B-lymphocytes and result in antibody production by plasma cells. Antibodies destroy the invading organism (usually in the extracellular compartment).

expression of these genes. Moreover, IL-1 and TNF act synergistically in this process. Figure 2 illustrates the basic events of an inflammatory process. Whether induced by infection, trauma, ischemia, immune-activated T cells, or toxins; IL-1 and TNF initiate the cascade of inflammatory mediators by targeting the endothelium.

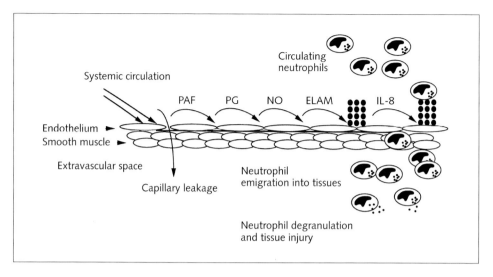

Figure 2
Pro-inflammatory effects of IL-1 and TNF are on the endothelium.
TNF and IL-1 activate endothelial cells and trigger the cascade of pro-inflammatory small molecule mediators. Increased gene expression for phospholipase A_2 type II, cyclooxygenase type-2 (COX-2) and inducible nitric oxide synthase (iNOS) results in elevated production of their products, PAF, PGE_2 and NO. Alone or in combination, these mediators decrease the tone of vascular smooth muscle. IL-1 and TNF also cause increased capillary leakage leading to swelling and pain. Pain thresholds are lowered by PGE_2. The upregulation of endothelial leukocyte adhesion molecules results in adherence of circulating neutrophils to the endothelium and increased production of chemokines such as IL-8 facilitates the migration of neutrophils into the tissues. Chemokines also activate degranulation of neutrophils. Activated neutrophils lead to tissue destruction and more inflammation.
PAF, platelet activating factor; PG, prostaglandin; NO, nitric oxide; ELAM, endothelial-leukocyte adhesion molecule; IL-8, interleukin-8

On the other hand, anti-inflammatory cytokines block this process or at least suppress the intensity of the cascade. Cytokines such as IL-4, IL-10, IL-13, and transforming growth factor β (TGFβ) suppress the production of IL-1, TNF, chemokines such as IL-8, and vascular adhesion molecules. Therefore, a "balance" between the effects of pro- and anti-inflammatory cytokines is thought to determine the outcome of disease, whether short or long term. In fact, some studies have data suggesting that susceptibility to disease is genetically determined by the balance or expression of either pro- or anti-inflammatory cytokines. Gene linkage studies are, however, often difficult to interpret. Nevertheless, deletion of the IL-10 gene in mice makes the animals vulnerable to the development of a fatal inflammatory bowel disease and similar studies have been reported for deletion of the IL-1 receptor antagonist (IL-1Ra) and TGFβ1 genes.

IL-1, TNF and pain

As shown in Table 2, synergism of IL-1 and TNF is a commonly reported phenomenon. Clearly, both cytokines are being produced at sites of local inflammation and hence the net effect should be considered when making correlations between cytokine levels and severity of disease. There is also synergism between IL-1 and bradykinin as well as IL-1 or TNF and mesenchymal growth factors. Most relevant to pain is the increase in PGE_2 stimulated by IL-1 or the combination of IL-1 and

Table 2 - Synergistic activities of IL-1 and TNF

IL-1 plus TNF	Hemodynamic shock and lactic acidosis in rabbits
	Radioprotection
	Generation of Shwartzman reaction
	Luteal cell $PGF_{2\alpha}$ synthesis
	PGE_2 synthesis in fibroblasts
	Galactosamine-induced hepatotoxicity
	Sickness behavior in mice
	Circulating nitric oxide and hypoglycemia in malaria
	Nerve growth factor synthesis from fibroblasts
	Insulin release and beta islet cell death
	Insulin resistance
	Loss of lean body mass
	IL-8 synthesis by mesothelial cells
IL-1 plus bradykinin	Angiogenesis
	PGE_2 synthesis in gingival fibroblasts
	Arachidonic acid release from synoviocytes
	$PGF_{2\alpha}$ synthesis in uterine decidua
	IL-6 production from hepatoma cells and fibroblasts
IL-1 or TNF plus FGF or PDGF or EGF or TGFα	PGE_2 synthesis in dermal fibroblasts
	PGE_2 synthesis in synovial cells
	Chemotaxis for fibroblasts
	Phospholipase A_2 release from synoviocytes
	Degradation of articular cartilage
	PGE_2 synthesis in osteoblastic cells

TNF. Although addressed in other chapters, IL-1 lowers the threshold to pain primarily by increasing PGE_2 synthesis [1].

If one examines the biological effects of IL-1 and asks the question: what is the most consistent property of IL-1? The answer would be: to increase the synthesis of PGE_2. In fact, the use of cyclooxygenase inhibitors for a variety of inflammatory conditions is often a therapeutic strategy to reduce IL-1-induced PGE_2. Humans injected with IL-1 experience fever, headache, myalgias, and arthralgias, each of which is reduced by co-administration of cyclooxygenase inhibitors [2]. One of the more universal activities of IL-1 is the induction of gene expression for type-II phospholipase A_2 and COX-2. IL-1 induces transcription of COX-2 and seems to have little effect on increased production of COX-1. Moreover, once triggered, COX-2 production is elevated for several hours and large amounts of PGE_2 are produced in cells stimulated with IL-1. Therefore, it comes as no surprise that many biological activities of IL-1 are actually due to increased PGE_2 production. Table 3 depicts cyclooxygenase dependent effects of IL-1 *in vitro* and *in vivo*.

There appears to be selectivity in cyclooxygenase inhibitors in that some non-steroidal anti-inflammatory agents are better inhibitors of COX-2 rather than COX-1. Similar to COX-2 induction, IL-1 preferentially stimulates new transcripts for the inducible type-II form of PLA_2 which cleaves the fatty acid in the number 2 position of cell membrane phospholipids. In most cases, this is arachidonic acid. The release of arachidonic acid is the rate limiting step in the synthesis of prostaglandins and leukotrienes. IL-1 also stimulates increased leukotriene synthesis in many cells.

One must consider that when cells are stimulated with IL-1 *in vitro*, a significant release of PGE_2 takes place and that, in the absence of cyclooxygenase inhibitors, PGE_2 accumulates in the culture vessel and exerts its own effects. For example, human smooth muscle cells incubated with IL-1 produce large amounts of PGE_2 which suppresses the proliferation of these cells; when cyclooxygenase inhibitors are incorporated into the culture, IL-1 stimulates cell proliferation [3]. Most genes induced by IL-1 are not affected by inhibiting PGE_2 synthesis. Gene expression of other cytokines, collagenases, colony stimulating factors and hepatic acute phase proteins are unaffected by cyclooxygenase inhibitors added to cultured cells or administered *in vivo*. On the other hand, many activities of IL-1 in the central nervous system are mediated by the formation of prostaglandins. IL-1 induction of sleep is an exception.

IL-1 receptors and signal transduction

Receptors
Both IL-1 forms (IL-1α and IL-1β), as well as IL-1Ra, have been found in the central nervous system and peripheral nervous tissues. In the brain, IL-1 appears in

Table 3 - Cyclooxygenase-dependent activities of IL-1

In vivo	Fever
	Natriuresis
	ACTH and growth hormone release
	Suppression of norepinephrine release
	Enhancement of capsaicin hyperemia
	Suppression of T cell mitogenesis
	Increased mucosal ion transport
	Colonic hypersecretion
	c-fos expression in brain
	Gastroparesis
	Decreased pain threshold
	Suppression of appetite and weight loss
	Suppression of insulin release
	Hyerinsulinemia
	Rapid arterial relaxation
	Hypotension in rabbits
	Edema, leukocyte infiltration and substance P after intra-articular Injection
	Increased melanoma bone marrow metastases
	Increased cerebrospinal calcium levels
	Decreased water intake
	Protection against: Hypoxic lung damage
	Skin hypersensitivity
	Inflammatory bowel disease
In vitro	Facilitation of ion-transport
	Suppression of smooth muscle cell proliferation[1]
	Inhibition of HLA-DR expression
	Increased corticotropin releasing factor
	Formation of osteoclasts
	Expression of heme oxygenase-1 gene expression
	Collagenase and stromelysin[2]
	Increased relaxation of arterial vessels
	Osteoblast production of IGF-I[3]
	Inhibition of bone mineralization
	Increased IGF-I production in bone cultures[3]
	Induction of LIF in fibroblasts[3]

[1] *IL-1-induced PGE_2 may augment gene expression and/or synthesis of some IL-1-induced genes, for example other cytokines and iNOS via increase cAMP*
[2] *IL-1 induced PGE effect is via increased cAMP formation.*
[3] *Co-injection of cyclooxygenase inhibitors augment the response*

microglia, glial cells, and in some studies in hypothalamic neurons [4]. Plata-Salaman has made extensive studies of the presence and regulation of IL-1 and IL-1R in the brain. The role of IL-1 and IL-1R in the brain substance is more relevant to events taking place in the central nervous system than in the periphery. This statement is based on the failure to demonstrate passage of IL-1 from the systemic circulation into the brain in a time-dependent fashion consistent with the event. For example, the intravenous injection of IL-1 produces fever, ACTH release and other hypothalamic events within minutes whereas during this time, no radiolabeled IL-1 can be found in hypothalamic centers. Several studies have provided data which suggest that IL-1 receptors are present on the specialized endothelial cells of the circumventricular organs or *organum vasculosum laminae terminalis* (OVLT).

These endothelial cells possess little if any blood-brain barrier. Ablation of the OVLT prevents fever after a peripheral injection of IL-1. It is likely that endothelial cells lining the OVLT respond to blood-borne IL-1 and release arachidonic acid metabolites. Metabolites of cyclooxygenase may then diffuse the few millimeters into the preoptic/anterior hypothalamic region and initiate fever. Alternatively, PGE_2 and other prostaglandins may be produced by the endothelial cells which, in turn, induce a neurotransmitter-like substance that acts to raise the set-point. This explanation is actually likely, since prostaglandins are not suitable as neurotransmitters. PGE_2 is known to increase levels of cyclic AMP, which has neurotransmitter properties in brain tissue, and has been implicated in fever and other central nervous system (CNS) pathways.

Two primary IL-1 binding proteins (receptors[R]) have been identified and one receptor accessory protein (IL-1R-AcP) [5, 6]. The extracellular domains of the two receptors and the IL-1R-AcP are members of the immunoglobulin superfamily, each comprising of three IgG-like domains and sharing a significant homology to each other. The two IL-1 receptors are distinct gene products and, in humans, the genes for IL-1RI and IL-1RII are located on the long arm of chromosome 2 [7].

IL-1RI is an 80 kDa glycoprotein found prominently on endothelial cells, smooth muscle cells, epithelial cells, hepatocytes, fibroblasts, keratinocytes, epidermal dendritic cells and T lymphocytes. IL-1RI is heavily glycosylated and blocking the glycosylation sites reduces the binding of IL-1 [8]. Surface expression of this receptor is likely on most IL-1-responsive cells as biological activity of IL-1 is a better assessment of receptor expression than ligand binding. Failure to show specific and saturable IL-1 binding is often due to the low numbers of surface IL-1RI on primary cells [9]. In cell lines, the number of IL-1RI can reach 5,000 per cell but primary cells usually express less that 200 receptors per cell. In some primary cells there are less than 50 per cell and IL-1 signal transduction has been observed in cells expressing less than 10 type I receptors per cell. Interestingly, the cytosolic domain of IL-1RI has a 45% amino acid homology with the cytosolic domain of the *Drosophila Toll* gene [10]. Toll is a transmembrane protein which acts like a receptor although the ligand for the Toll protein is unknown. Gene organisation and amino acid homology suggests that the IL-1RI and the cytosolic Toll are derived from a common ancestor and trigger similar signals [11].

Like other models of two chain receptors, IL-1 binds first to the IL-1RI with a low affinity. The crystal structure of the IL-1RI complexed with IL-1β has been reported and sheds light on the changes that take place after the low affinity binding [12]. The two receptor binding sites of IL-1β have been reported using specific mutations. The crystal structure reveals that both receptor binding sites contact the IL-1RI at the first and third domains [12]. Upon contact with the first domain, there appears to be a change in the rigidity of the third domain enabling contact with the second binding site of IL-1β. IL-1β itself does not undergo a structural change. IL-1Ra has only one binding site [13] and absence of the second binding site prevents contact with the third domain. Hence, the critical contact point appears to be

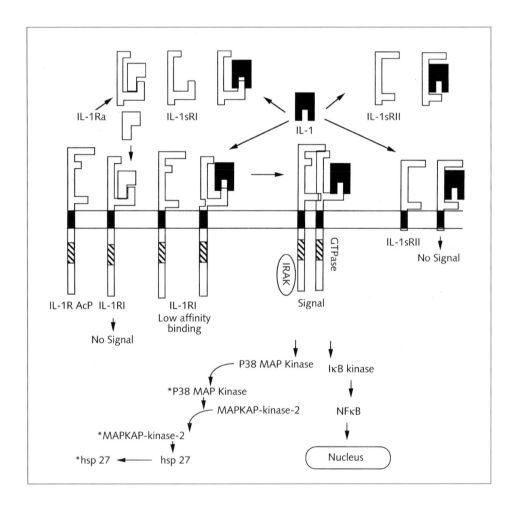

at the third domain. Since this contact is likely to be absent in complexes with the IL-1Ra [14], the structural change in the IL-1RI third domain may allow docking of the IL-1R-AcP with the IL-1RI/IL-1β complex. Without the complex of IL-1R-AcP/IL-1RI/IL-1β, there is no signal transduction [6]. Figure 3 illustrates the relationship of IL-1 binding to its receptor and triggering post-receptor events.

Antibodies to the type I receptor and to the IL-1R-AcP block IL-1 binding and activity [6]. The IL-1R-AcP is essential to IL-1 signaling; in cells deficient in IL-1R-AcP, no IL-1-induced activation of the stress kinases takes place but this response is restored upon transfection with a construct expressing the IL-1R-AcP [15]. Affinity-purified antibodies to the IL-1R-AcP third domain amino acids preferentially block IL-1β activity [16] suggesting that the docking of the IL-1R-AcP with the IL-1RI takes place with the third domain of each receptor.

Figure 3
An IL-1 responsive cell.
In this model, IL-1 is shown. IL-1 binds to the extracellular domain of either type I (IL-1RI) or type II (IL-1RII). Although there is preferential binding of IL-1β to IL-1RII, this receptor, lacking a cytosolic segment, does not transduce a signal but rather acts as a decoy receptor or a "sink" for IL-1β. Following low affinity binding of IL-1β to the IL-1RI, there is a structural change in the third IgG-like domain of this receptor. This structural change allows for the IL-1R accessory protein (IL-1RAcP) to form a compex with the low affinity IL-1/IL-1RI. This results in a high affinity complex (IL-1R-AcP/IL-1/IL-1RI) and in signal transduction. Lacking a second binding site, IL-1 receptor antagonist (IL-1Ra) binds primarily to IL-1RI but does not result in a structural change in the receptor. Hence the IL-1R-AcP does not form a high affinity complex with the IL-1/IL-1R, no signal is transduced and there is no biological response. Signal transduction appears to require the formation of a heterodimer of IL-1RI with IL-1R-AcP. The cytoplasmic domain of the IL-1RI contains areas with putative GTPase activity. Proteins associating with the IL-1RI cytoplasmic domains include a GTPase activating protein and the IL-1R activating kinase (IRAK) which is recruited by the IL-1R-AcP. Cells expressing receptors for IL-1RII compete with the binding of IL-1 to the cell bound receptors of IL-1RI and in those cells with excess IL-1RII a reduced biological response to IL-1 is thought to take place.
IL-1 may also bind to soluble receptors found in the circulation and extracellular fluids. There is a hierachy of binding to these soluble receptors. The soluble extracellular domain of IL-1RI (IL-1sRI) binds IL-1Ra > IL-1α > IL-1β; the soluble part of the extracellular domain of IL-1RII (IL-1sRII) binds IL-1β > proIL-1β > IL-1α > IL-1Ra. Ten-fold molar excesses of IL-1sRII and IL-1sRI over IL-1 and IL-1Ra, respectively, usually exist in the circulation of healthy subjects. Nevertheless, dramatic responses to intravenously injected IL-1 take place and hence the affinity of these soluble receptors must be less than that of the cell-bound receptors.

IL-1 decoy receptor

IL-1RII has a short cytosolic domain consisting of 29 amino acids. This type II receptor appears to act as a "decoy" molecule, particularly for IL-1β. The receptor binds IL-1β tightly thus preventing binding to the signal transducing type I receptor [17]. It is the lack of a signal transducing cytosolic domain which makes the type II receptor a functionally negative receptor. For example, when the extracellular portion of the type II receptor is fused to the cytoplasmic domain of the type I receptor, a biological signal occurs [18]. The extracellular portion of the type II receptor is found in body fluids where it is termed IL-1 soluble receptor type II (IL-1sRII). It is assumed that a proteolytic cleavage of the extracelluar domain of the IL-1RII from the cell surface is the source of the IL-1sRII.

It is likely that as cell bound IL-1RII increases, there is a comparable increase in soluble forms [19]. Similar to soluble receptors for TNF, the extracellular domain of the type I and type II IL-1R are found as "soluble" molecules in the circulation and urine of healthy subjects and in inflammatory synovial and other pathological body fluids [20–22]. In healthy humans, the circulating levels of IL-1sRII are 100-200 pM whereas levels of IL-1sRI are 10-fold less. The rank of affinities for the two soluble receptors are remarkably different for each of the three IL-1 molecules. The rank for the three IL-1 ligands binding to IL-1sRI is IL-1Ra > IL-1α > IL-1β whereas for IL-1sRII the rank is IL-1β > IL-1α > IL-1Ra. Elevated levels of IL-1sRII are found in the circulation of patients with sepsis [23] and in the synovial fluid of patients with active rheumatoid arthritis [22] whereas the elevations of soluble type I receptor in these fluids are 10-fold lower.

Unlike other cytokines receptors, in cells expressing both IL-1 type I and type II receptors, there is competition to bind IL-1 first. This competition between signaling and non-signaling receptors for the same ligand appears unique to cytokine receptors, although it exists for atrial natriuretic factor receptors. Since the type II receptor is more likely to bind to IL-1β than IL-1α, this can result in a diminished response to IL-1β. The soluble form of IL-1sRII circulates in healthy humans at molar concentrations which are 10-fold greater than those of IL-1β measured in septic patients and 100-fold greater than the concentration of IL-1β following intravenous administration [24, 25]. Why do humans have a systemic response to an infusion of IL-1β? One concludes that binding of IL-1β to the soluble form of IL-1R type II exhibits a slow "on" rate compared to the cell IL-1RI.

Signal transduction

Within a few minutes following binding to cells, IL-1 induces several biochemical events (reviewed in [26–29]). It remains unclear which is the most "upstream" triggering event or whether several occur at the same time. No sequential order or cascade has been identified but several signaling events appear to be taking place during the first 2–5 minutes. Some of the biochemical changes associated with signal transduction are likely to be cell specific. Within two minutes, hydrolysis of GTP, phosphotidylcholine, phosphotidylserine or phosphotidylethanolamine [30, 31] and release of ceramide by neutral [32] (not acidic) sphingomyelinase [33] have been reported. In general, multiple protein phosphorylations and activation of phosphatases can be observed within five minutes [34] and some are thought to be initiated by the release of lipid mediators. The release of ceramide has attracted attention as a possible early signaling event [35]. Phosphorylation of PLA_2 activating protein also occurs in the first few minutes [36] which would lead to a rapid release of arachidonic acid. Multiple and similar signaling events have also been reported for TNF.

With few exceptions, there is general agreement that IL-1 does not stimulate hydrolysis of phosphatidylinositol or an increase in intracellular calcium. Without a clear increase in intracellular calcium, early post-receptor binding events nevertheless include hydrolysis of a GTP with no associated increase in adenyl cyclase, activation of adenyl cyclase [37, 38], hydrolysis of phospholipids [9, 39], release of ceramide [40] and release of arachidonic acid from phopholipids via cytosolic phospholipase A_2 (PLA_2) following its activation by PLA_2 activating protein [36]. Some IL-1 signaling events are prominent in different cells. Post-receptor signaling mechanisms may therefore provide cellular specificity. For example, in some cells, IL-1 is a growth factor and signaling is associated with serine/threonine phosphorylation of the MAP kinase p42/44 in mesangial cells [41]. The MAP p38 kinase, another member of the MAP kinase family, is phosphorylated in fibroblasts [42], as is the p54α MAP kinase in hepatocytes [43].

The cytoplasmic domain of IL-1RI does not contain a consensus sequence for intrinsic tyrosine phosphorylation but deletion mutants of the receptor reveal specific functions for some domains. There are four nuclear localization sequences which share homology with the glucocorticoid receptor. Three amino acids (Arg-431, Lys-515 and Arg-518), also found in the Toll protein, are essential for IL-1-induced IL-2 production [11]. However, deletion of a segment containing these amino acids did not affect IL-1-induced IL-8 [44]. There are also two cytoplasmic domains in the IL-1RI which share homology with the IL-6-signaling gp130 receptor. When these regions are deleted, there is a loss of IL-1-induced IL-8 production [44].

The C-terminal 30 amino acids of the IL-1RI can be deleted without affecting biological activity [45]. Two independent studies have focused on the area between amino acids 513-529. Amino acids 508-521 contain sites required for the activation of NFκB. In one study, deletion of this segment abolished IL-1-induced IL-8 expression and in another study, specific mutations of amino acids 513 and 520 to alanine prevented IL-1-driven E-selectin promoter activity. This area is also present in the Toll protein domain associated with NFκB translocation and previously shown to be part of the IL-1 signaling mechanism. This area (513-520) is also responsible for activating a kinase which associates with the receptor. This kinase, termed "IL-1 receptor associated kinase" or IRAK, phosphorylates a 100 kDa substrate [45]. IRAK is thought to phosphorylate the NFκB kinase (NIK) which leads to degradation of IκB. As shown previously, IL-1 degrades IκB [46]. Thus, following receptor binding, the IL-1R-AcP recruits IRAK, which leads to degradation of IκB and translocation of NFκB to the nucleus. However, downstream events and activation of other transcriptions factors such as AP-1 and tyrosine phosphorylation of MAP kinases also take place.

IL-1 receptor binding results in the phosphorylation of tyrosine residues [42, 43]. Tyrosine phosphorylation induced by IL-1 is likely due to activation of MAP kinase which then phosphorylates tyrosine and threonine on MAP kinases. Following activation of MAP kinases, there are phosphorylations on serine and threonine residues of the epidermal growth factor receptor, heat-shock protein p27, myelin basic protein and serine 56 and 156 of β-casein, each of which has been observed in IL-1-stimulated cells [47]; TNF also activates these kinases. There are at least three families of MAP kinases. The p42/44 MAP kinase family is associated with signal transduction by growth factors including ras-raf-1 signal pathways. In rat mesangial cells, IL-1 activates the p42/44 MAP kinase within ten minutes and also increases *de novo* synthesis of p42 [41].

In addition to p42/44, two members of the MAP kinase family (p38 and p54) have been identified as part of an IL-1 phosphorylation pathway and are responsible for phosphorylating heat shock protein (hsp) 27 [42, 43]. These MAP kinases are highly conserved proteins homologous to the *HOG-1* stress gene in yeasts. In fact, when *HOG-1* is deleted, yeasts fail to grow in hyperosmotic conditions; however, the mammalian gene coding for the IL-1-inducible p38 MAP kinase [43] can reconstitute the ability of the yeast to grow in hyperosmotic conditions [48]. In cells stimulated with hyperosmolar NaCl, LPS, IL-1 or TNF, indistinguishable phosphorylation of the p38 MAP kinase takes place [49]. In human monocytes exposed to hyperosmolar NaCl (375–425 milliosmoles/l), IL-8, IL-1β, IL-1α and TNFα gene expression and synthesis takes place which is indistinguishable from that induced by LPS or IL-1 [50, 51]. Thus, the MAP p38 kinase pathways involved in IL-1, TNF and LPS signal transductions share certain elements that are related to the primitive stress-induced pathway.

IL-1-induces several transcription factors. Most of the biological effects of IL-1 take place in cells following nuclear translocation of NFκB and activating protein-1 (AP-1), two nuclear factors common to many IL-1-induced genes. In T lymphocytes and cultured hepatocytes, the addition of IL-1 increases nuclear binding of c-jun and c-fos, the two components of AP-1 [52]. Similar to NFκB, AP-1 sites are present in the promoter regions of many IL-1-inducible genes. IL-1 also increases the transcription of *c-jun* by activating two novel nuclear factors (jun-1 and jun-2) which bind to the promoter of the *c-jun* gene and stimulate *c-jun* transcription [53].

How does IL-1 differ from TNF in activating cells?

From the above descriptions of IL-1R and IL-1 signal transduction, many of these pathways are shared with TNF. Although the receptors for TNF and IL-1 are clearly different, the post-receptor events are amazingly similar. Thus, the finding that IL-1 and TNF activate the same portfolio of genes is not surprising. However, given the same cell and given the same array of activated genes, IL-1 does not result in programmed cell death whereas TNF does. This can be seen in TNF responsive fibroblasts in which IL-1 and TNF induce IL-8 but in the presence of actinomycin C (which disrupts transcription) or cycloheximide (which disrupts protein synthesis), TNF induces classical apoptosis but IL-1 does not. IL-1 will often synergize with TNF for nitric oxide induction and under these conditions, nitric oxide mediates cell death. The best example of this can be found in the insulin-producing beta cells in the islets of Langerhans in the pancreas [54]. Unlike IL-1, the receptors for TNF are homodimers and trimers and hence the recruitment of kinases is somewhat different. However, the cytosolic domain of the TNF p55 receptor contains a "death domain" which recruits intracellular molecules involved with initiating programmed cell death [55]. There is no comparable "death domain" in the cytoplasmic domains of either the IL-1RI or the IL-1R-AcP.

There are two receptors for TNF, the p55 receptor and the p75 receptor [56]. Although TNF binds and triggers both receptors, the cytosolic domains of these receptors recruit different proteins which transduce the TNF signal further. In one case, the p55 receptor cytosolic domain is linked to pathways of cell death whereas the p75 is not. Both receptors, however, result in the translocation of the nuclear factor B (NFκB) to the nucleus where it binds to the promoter regions of a variety of genes. These gene products are often the same as those triggered by IL-1 which also results in translocation of NFκB to the nucleus. The difference is, however, that the cytosolic domains of the p55 tumor necrosis factor receptor (TNFR) are unique in their ability to activate intracellular signals leading to programmed cell death (also called apoptosis). The p55 TNFR has the so-called "death domain" and recruits a protein called MORT-1. Also involved in this process are a family of intracellular proteins which become activated and are called TRAFs for "TNF receptor associated factors". Presently there are 6 or perhaps 8 TRAFs. The p55 cytosolic domains also recruit the family of intracellular proteins called TRADDs (TNF receptor associated death domains). Overexpression of TRADDs results in cell death and activation of NFκB. TRADDs also lead to activation of the caspase family of intracellular cysteine proteases. Although caspase-1 (also known as the IL-1β converting enzyme, ICE) is important for processing the precursors for proIL-1β and proIL-18, other members of this family are also part of the TNF cell death signaling pathway.

One interesting aspect of the biology of TNF in the brain is the ability of TNF to both protect neurons as well as to initiate their self destruction. Both pathways involve activation of NFκB [57]. In general, the state of the cell (cell cycle) may help explain why activation of NFκB can be associated with both protection from cell death as well as apoptosis. One is reminded that activation of NFκB leads most often to new protein synthesis; some proteins from this process are clearly inducing cell proliferation whereas others induce cell death.

Acknowledgement
Supported by NIH Grant AI-15614

References

1   Schweizer A, Feige U, Fontana A, Muller K, Dinarello CA (1988) Interleukin-1 enhances pain reflexes. Mediation through increased prostaglandin E$_2$ levels. *Agents Actions* 25: 246–251

2   Janik JE, Miller LL, Longo DL, Powers GC, Urba WJ, Kopp WC, Gause BL, Curti BD, Fenton RG, Oppenheim JJ, Conlon KC, Holmlund JT, Sznol M, Sharfman WH, Steis RG, Creekmore SP, Alvord WG, Beauchamp AE, Smith JW 2nd (1996) Phase II trial of interleukin 1 alpha and indomethacin in treatment of metastatic melanoma. *J Natl Cancer Inst* 88: 44–49

3   Libby P, Warner SJ, Friedman GB (1988) Interleukin 1: a mitogen for human vascular smooth muscle cells that induces the release of growth-inhibitory prostanoids. *J Clin Invest* 81: 487–498

4   Breder CD, Dinarello CA, Saper CB (1988) Interleukin-1 immunoreactive innervation of the human hypothalamus. *Science* 240: 321–324

5   Sims JE, Giri JG, Dower SK (1994) The two interleukin-1 receptors play different roles in IL-1 activities. *Clin Immunol Immunopathol* 72: 9–14

6   Greenfeder SA, Nunes P, Kwee L, Labow M, Chizzonite RA, Ju G (1995) Molecular cloning and characterization of a second subunit of the interleukin-1 receptor complex. *J Biol Chem* 270: 13757–13765

7   Sims JE, Painter SL, Gow IR (1995) Genomic organization of the type I and type II IL-1 receptors. *Cytokine* 7: 483–490

8   Mancilla J, Ikejima I, Dinarello CA (1992) Glycosylation of the interleukin-1 receptor type I is required for optimal binding of interleukin-1. *Lymphokine Cytokine Res* 11: 197–205

9   Rosoff PM, Savage N, Dinarello CA (1988) Interleukin-1 stimulates diacylglycerol production in T lymphocytes by a novel mechanism. *Cell* 54: 73–81

10   Gay NJ, Keith FJ (1991) *Drosophila Toll* and IL-1 receptor. *Nature* 351: 355–356

11   Heguy A, Baldari CT, Macchia G, Telford JL, Melli M (1992) Amino acids conserved in interleukin-1 receptors and the Drosophila Toll protein are essential for IL-1R signal transduction. *J Biol Chem* 267: 2605–2609

12   Vigers GPA, Anderson LJ, Caffes P, Brandhuber BJ (1997) Crystal structure of the type I interleukin-1 receptor complexed with interleukin-1β. *Nature* 386: 190–194

13   Evans RJ, Bray J, Childs JD, Vigers GP, Brandhuber BJ, Skalicky JJ, Thompson RC, Eisenberg SP (1995) Mapping receptor binding sites in interleukin (IL)-1 receptor antagonist and IL-1 beta by site-directed mutagenesis: identification of a single site in IL-1ra and two sites in IL-1 beta. *J Biol Chem* 270 (19): 11477–11483

14   Schreuder H, Tardif C, Trump-Kallmeyer S, Soffientini A, Sarubbi E, Akeson A, Bowlin T, Yanofsky S, Barrett RW (1997) A new cytokine-receptor binding mode revealed by the crystal structure of the IL-1 receptor with an antagonist. *Nature* 386 (6621): 194–200

15   Wesche H, Korherr C, Kracht M, Falk W, Resch K, Martin MU (1997) The interleukin-1 receptor accessory protein is essential for IL-1-induced activation of interleukin-1 receptor-associated kinase (IRAK) and stress-activated protein kinases (SAP kinases). *J Biol Chem* 272: 7727–7731

16   Yoon D-Y, Dinarello CA (1996) Regulation of IL-1 receptor tyep I and accessory protein by IL-10. *Eur Cytokine Netw* 7: 547 (abs)

17   Colotta F, Re F, Muzio M, Bertini R, Polentarutti N, Sironi M, Giri JG, Dower SK, Sims JE, Mantovani A (1993) Interleukin-1 type II receptor: a decoy target for IL-1 that is regulated by IL-4. *Science* 261: 472–475

18   Heguy A, Baldari CT, Censini S, Ghiara P, Telford JL (1993) A chimeric type II/I interleukin-1 receptor can mediate interleukin-1 induction of gene expression in T cells. *J Biol Chem* 268: 10490–10494

19   Giri J, Newton RC, Horuk R (1990) Identification of soluble interleukin-1 binding protein in cell-free supernatants. *J Biol Chem* 265: 17416–17419

20   Symons JA, Eastgate JA, Duff GW (1991) Purification and characterization of a novel soluble receptor for interleukin-1. *J Exp Med* 174: 1251–1254

21   Symons JA, Young PA, Duff GW (1993) The soluble interleukin-1 receptor: ligand binding properties and mechanisms of release. *Lymphokine Cytokine Res* 12: 381

22   Arend WP, Malyak M, Smith MF Jr, Whisenand TD, Slack JL, Sims JE, Giri JG, Dower SK (1994) Binding of IL-1 alpha, IL-1 beta, and IL-1 receptor antagonist by soluble IL-1 receptors and levels of soluble IL-1 receptors in synovial fluids. *J Immunol* 153 (10): 4766–4774

23   Giri JG, Wells J, Dower SK, McCall CE, Guzman RN, Slack J, Bird TA, Shanebeck K, Grabstein KH, Sims JE (1994) Elevated levels of shed type II IL-1 receptor in sepsis. Potential role for type ll receptor in regulation of IL-1 responses. *J Immunol* 153 (12): 5802–5809

24   Crown J, Jakubowski A, Kemeny N, Gordon M, Gasparetto C, Wong G, Sheridan C, Toner G, Meisenberg B, Botet J (1991) A phase I trial of recombinant human interleukin-1 beta alone and in combination with myelosuppressive doses of 5-fluoruracil in patients with gastrointestinal cancer. *Blood* 78 (6): 1420–1427

25   Crown J, Jakubowski A, Gabrilove J (1993) Interleukin-1: biological effects in human hematopoiesis. *Leuk Lymphoma* 9: 433–440

26 O'Neill LAJ (1995) Towards an understanding of the signal transduction pathways for interleukin-1. *Biochim Biophys Acta* 1266: 31–44

27 Mizel SB (1994) IL-1 signal transduction. *Eur Cytokine Netw* 5: 547–561

28 Rossi B (1993) IL-1 transduction signals. *Eur Cytokine Netw* 4: 181–187

29 Kuno K, Matsushima K (1994) The IL-1 receptor signaling pathway. *J Leukoc Biol* 56: 542–547

30 Rosoff PM (1990) IL-1 receptors: structure and signals. *Seminars in Immunology* 2:129–137

31 Rosoff PM (1989) Characterization of the interleukin-1-stimulated phospholipase C activity in human T lymphocytes. *Lymphokine Res* 8: 407–413

32 Schutze S, Machleidt T, Kronke M (1994) The role of diacylglycerol and ceramide in tumor necrosis factor and interleukin-1 signal transduction. *J Leukoc Biol* 56: 533–541

33 Andrieu N, Salvayre R, Levade T (1994) Evidence against involvement of the acid lysosomal sphingomyelinase in the tumor necrosis factor and interleukin-1-induced sphingomyelin cycle and cell proliferation in human fibroblasts. *Biochem J* 303: 341–345

34 Bomalaski JS, Steiner MR, Simon PL, Clark MA (1992) IL-1 increases phospholipase A2 activity, expression of phospholipase A_2-activating protein, and release of linoleic acid from the murine T helper cell line EL-4. *J Immunol* 148: 155–160

35 Kolesnick R, Golde DW (1994) The sphingomyelin pathway in tumor necrosis factor and interleukin-1 signalling. *Cell* 77: 325–328

36 Gronich J, Konieczkowski M, Gelb MH, Nemenoff RA, Sedor JR (1994) Interleukin-1α causes a rapid activation of cytosolic phospholipase A_2 by phosphorylation in rat mesangial cells. *J Clin Invest* 93: 1224–1233

37 Mizel SB (1990) Cyclic AMP and interleukin-1 signal transduction. *Immunol Today* 11: 390–391

38 Munoz E, Beutner U, Zubiaga A, Huber BT (1990) IL-1 activates two separate signal transduction pathways in T helper type II cells. *J Immunol* 144: 964–969

39 Kester M, Siomonson MS, Mene P, Sedor JR (1989) Interleukin-1 generate transmembrane signals from phospholipids through novel pathways in cultured rat mesangial cells. *J Clin Invest* 83: 718–723

40 Mathias S, Younes A, Kan C-C, Orlow I, Joseph C, Kolesnick RN (1993) Activation of the sphingomyelin signaling pathway in intact EL4 cells and in a cell-free system by IL-1β. *Science* 259: 519–522

41 Huwiler A, Pfeilschifter J (1994) Interleukin-1 stimulates de novo synthesis of mitogen-activated protein kinase in glomerular mesangial cells. *FEBS Lett* 350: 135–138

42 Freshney NW, Rawlinson L, Guesdon F, Jones E, Cowley S, Hsuan J, Saklatvala J (1994) Interleukin-1 activates a novel protein kinase cascade that results in the phosphorylation of hsp27. *Cell* 78 (6): 1039–1049

43 Kracht M, Truong O, Totty NF, Shiroo M, Saklatvala J (1994) Interleukin-1α activates two forms of p54α mitogen-activated proetin kinase in rabbit liver. *J Exp Med* 180: 2017–2027

44 Kuno K, Okamoto S, Hirose K, Murakami S, Matsushima K (1993) Structure and func-

tion of the intracellular portion of the mouse interleukin-1 receptor (Type I). *J Biol Chem* 268: 13510–13518

45   Croston GE, Cao Z, Goeddel DV (1995) NFκB activation by interleukin-1 requires an IL-1 receptor-associated protein kinase activity. *J Biol Chem* 270: 16514–16517

46   DiDonato JA, Mercurio F, Karin M (1995) Phosphorylation of IκBα precedes but is not sufficient for its dissociation from NFκB. *Mol Cell Biol* 15: 1302–1311

47   Bird TA, Sleath PR, de Roos PC, Dower SK, Virca GD (1991) Interleukin-1 represents a new modality for the activation of extracellular signal-related kinases/microtubule-associated protein-2 kinases. *J Bio Chem* 266: 22661–22670

48   Galcheva-Gargova Z, Dérijard B, Wu I-H, Davis RJ (1994) An osmosensing signal transduction pathway in mammalian cells. *Science* 265: 806–809

49   Han J, Lee J-D, Bibbs L, Ulevitch RJ (1994) A MAP kinase targeted by endotoxin and hyperosmolarity in mammalian cells. *Science* 265: 808–811

50   Shapiro L, Dinarello CA (1997) Cytokine expression during osmotic stress. *Exp Cell Res* 231: 354–362

51   Shapiro L, Dinarello CA (1995) Osmotic regulation of cytokine synthesis *in vitro*. *Proc Natl Acad Sci USA* 92: 12230–12234

52   Muegge K, Williams TM, Kant J, Karin M, Chiu R, Schmidt A, Siebenlist U, Young HA, Durum SK (1989) Interleukin-1 costimulatory activity on the interleukin-2 promoter via AP-1. *Science* 246 (4927): 249–251

53   Muegge K, Vila M, Gusella GL, Musso T, Herrlich P, Stein B, Durum SK (1993) IL-1 induction of the c-jun promoter. *Proc Natl Acad Sci USA* 90 (15): 7054–7058

54   Reimers JI, Bjerre U, Mandrup-Poulsen T, Nerup J (1994) Interleukin-1β induces diabetes and fever in normal rats by nitric oxide via induction of different nitric oxide synthases. *Cytokine* 6: 512–520

55   Boldin MP, Varfolomeev EE, Pancer Z, Mett IL, Camonis JH, Wallach D (1995) A novel protein that interacts with thr death domain of Fas/APO1 contains a sequence motif related to the death domain. *J Biol Chem* 270: 7795–7798

56   Engelmann H, Novick D, Wallach D (1990) Two tumor necrosis factor-binding proteins purified from human urine. Evidence for immunological cross-reactivity with cell surface tumor necrosis factor receptors. *J Biol Chem* 265: 1531–1536

57   van Antwerp DJ, Martin SJ, Vermna IM, Green DR (1998) Inhibition of TNF-induced apoptosis by NFκB. *Trends Cell Biol* 8: 107–111

Evolutionary perspectives of cytokines in pain

Andrea L. Clatworthy

Department of Integrative Biology and Pharmacology, University of Texas – Houston Medical School, 6431 Fannin, Houston, TX 77030, USA

Evolutionary aspects of nociception

It is clear that the ability of an animal to detect and react appropriately to an aversive stimulus is of fundamental importance to its survival. This ability is as important to invertebrates as it is to vertebrates, a fact that is underscored by behavioral evidence for the display of nociceptive behaviors in invertebrates (reviewed in [1, 2]. For example, locomotion away from a noxious stimulus has been observed in the simplest animals (see Fig. 1) including protozoans [3], flatworms [4] and jellyfish [5]. Anemones (Anthozoa) display relatively sophisticated, nociceptive behaviors that can be modified by aversive environmental stimuli [6, 7]. Anthozoa have among the simplest nervous systems in the animal kingdom and it has been postulated that the first functional nociceptive responses are likely to have occurred in this group. The nociceptive behaviors of the more advanced invertebrate, the marine mollusc *Aplysia californica*, and their modification by a variety of stimuli have been studied extensively over the last two decades. *Aplysia* display a variety of nociceptive behaviors in response to noxious mechanical or electrical stimulation including local body withdrawal, ink and opaline release, and escape locomotion [8]. The relative simplicity and accessibility of the *Aplysia* nervous system for intracellular recording make it a very attractive model system to understand neuronal correlations underlying these nociceptive behaviors and their modification. Consequently *Aplysia* has emerged as a useful model system to understand fundamental mechanisms underlying nociceptive plasticity and it will be the focus of this review. It has been suggested that general similarities between patterns of nociceptive behavior observed in *Aplysia* and more complex animals (e.g. rats and humans) represent common behavioral adaptions to ubiquitous selection pressures such as escape from a source of bodily injury and optimization of recuperation [2].

Cytokines and Pain, edited by Linda R. Watkins and Steven F. Maier
© 1999 Birkhäuser Verlag Basel/Switzerland

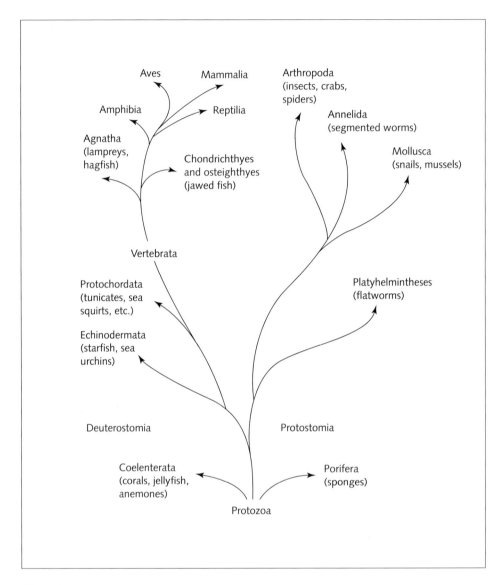

Figure 1
Phylogenetic tree illustrating the relationship between the main groups in the animal king-
dom. The two main divisions (Deuterostomia and Protostomia) are based upon differences
in embryological development. The branch on the left shows the development of the
deuterosomes – animals which eventually lead to the vertebrates. Note that echinoderms
and tunicates are deuterostome invertebrates. The right branch shows the development of
the protostomes. More than 95% of all extant animal species are protostome invertebrates.
Molluscs are protostome invertebrates. Modified after [31].

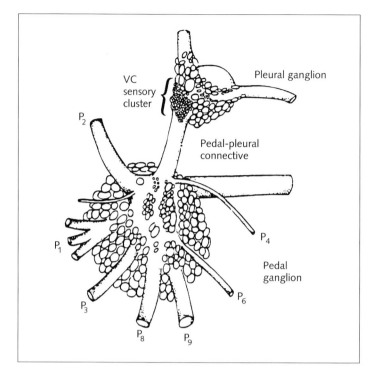

Figure 2
Schematic diagram of the Aplysia *left pleural and pedal ganglia. Symmetrical clusters of neurons are located in the contralateral (right) pleural-pedal ganglia. Ventro caudal (VC) pleural sensory cells located in the VC sensory cluster have large cell bodies (30–40 μm) that are easily accessible for intracellular recording. Each sensory cell sends a single axon out to the periphery through a specific, ipsilateral pedal nerve. Modified after [9].*

Nociceptive information processing in *Aplysia*

The central nervous system of *Aplysia* is distributed across ten major ganglia, each comprising 1,000 to 10,000 nerve cell bodies and many more glial support cells. A population of mechanosensory neurons located in the pleural ganglion in *Aplysia* have recently been identified as wide dynamic range nociceptors [9, 10]. These sensory cells (the VC pleural sensory cells: Fig. 2) that innervate the tail and most of the body wall (excluding the siphon) respond weakly to light pressure, but they show increasing discharges to increasing pressure with the maximal response evident following damaging or potentially damaging stimuli [10]. The response properties of these nociceptive sensory cells can be either enhanced or inhibited by noxious stimulation which is suggestive of a surprisingly complex degree of plasticity [10–13]. Indeed, detailed analysis of cellular mechanisms underlying nociceptive information processing in *Aplysia* has revealed remarkable similarities to mammalian species [14, 15].

Nociceptive sensory neurons in *Aplysia* undergo both transient and long-term alterations in their electrophysiological properties following noxious stimulation. For example, repetitive application of a noxious stimulus delivered to either a nerve or the skin leads to a progressive increase (wind-up) in the responses of nociceptive sensory neurons [10]. Figure 3 illustrates wind-up of discharge in a nociceptive tail sensory neuron in *Aplysia* in response to repeated administration of an electrical stimulus to the tail. Similarly, in mammalian preparations, repetitive application of a noxious stimulus or repeated nerve shock at c fibre strength leads to wind up of nociceptive neurons in the spinal cord and a consequent increase in pain [16, 17].

Body wall injury in *Aplysia* is also associated with profound long-term alterations in the electrophysiological properties of nociceptive sensory neurons. For example, brief, noxious stimulation of the skin of *Aplysia* can produce long lasting site-specific behavioral sensitization that is restricted to the region surrounding the damaged tissue [18]. Site-specific sensitization is associated with long lasting central and peripheral alterations in the population of sensory neurons that innervate the injured site [19]. Peripheral regions of sensory neurons innervating the damaged tissue exhibit a decrease in threshold and an increase in the number of action potentials evoked by a cutaneous test stimulus. The enhancement of central excitability is evidenced by a decrease in soma action potential threshold, a tendency for the soma to fire in regenerative bursts in response to a brief intracellular depolarizing stimulus and an enhancement of synaptic connections to identified motor neurons. This sensory plasticity appears to be mediated in part by a combination of intense spike activity in the sensory neuron having an axon in the injured region and exposure to neuromodulators released from nearby neurons [19]. Similar profound activity-dependent alterations in sensory processing are associated with primary hyperalgesia in mammalian preparations [2, 14].

More recently it has been found that profound long lasting increases in nociceptive sensory soma excitability and synaptic transmission can be produced by axonal injury in *Aplysia* under anaesthetic conditions where spike activity and neuromodulator release are largely blocked at the time of injury [20, 21]. This suggests that additional signals must be involved in mediating the injury-induced sensory hyperexcitability under these conditions. Compared to sensory neurons that did not have crushed axons, sensory cells with crushed axons had a significantly lower spike threshold and afterhyperpolarization, a significant increase in spike duration and a significant increase in the number of action potentials evoked by a standard 1 sec intracellular depolarizing pulse. There is delay in the expression of sensory hyperexcitability that is related to the distance of the crush site from the soma, and

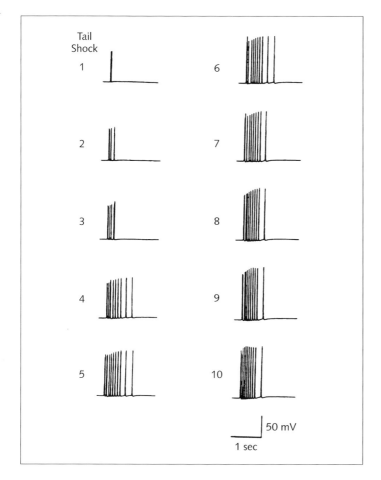

Figure 3
Wind-up of discharge in a nociceptive tail sensory neuron in Aplysia in response to repeated tail shock. A single 500 msec shock at four times the intensity to elicit a single spike was delivered ten times at 5 sec intervals. Reprinted with permission from [10].

inhibitors of retrogade transport prevent crush-induced sensory hyperexcitability [22]. These findings support the hypothesis that at least some of the signals initiating sensory hyperexcitability following crush are generated at the site of injury and transported to the soma via slow retrograde axonal transport. Potential signals include release of substances from damaged neurons or support cells, and release of factors from immune cells that are attracted to the site of crush (Fig. 4). Interestingly, blocking axonal transport by topical colchicine prevents hyperalgesia in a rat

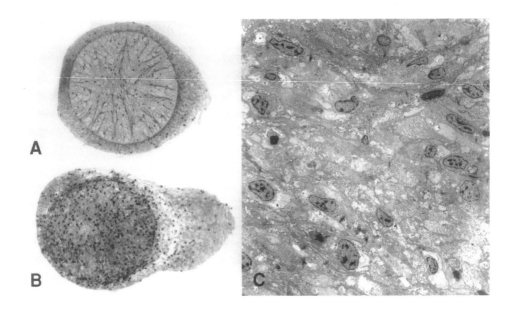

Figure 4
Light (A, B) and electron (C) microscopic views of cross sections through control (A), and crushed (B, C) pedal nerves 1 day after unilateral pedal nerve crush. There are few cells (black dots) associated with the control, uncrushed nerve section. In contrast, note the large accumulation of cells associated with the nerve section just distal to the crush site. The higher power electron micrograph (C) of a section through the crushed nerve illustrated in (B) shows that the cells associated with the crush site are hemocytes. Vesicles located in the cytoplasm contain dense material that resemble phagocytic vesicles characteristic of hemocytes. Reprinted with permission from [32].

model of neuropathic pain suggesting that factors generated at a site of injury are necessary for the development of neuropathic hyperalgersia [23].

Immune-mediated modulation of nociceptive processing

Recently, the involvement of the immune system in nociception has received much attention. In particular the influence of cytokines on nociceptive processing has been targeted. Studies have revealed a high degree of complexity. For example, IL-1β and tumor necrosis factor α (TNFα) have both been implicated in the induction of hyperalgesia following the administration of illness-inducing substances such as lipopolysaccharide (LPS) and lithium chloride [24]. Also, responses of afferent fibres to mechanical and thermal stimulation of the hind paw are enhanced by administration of a plantar injection of IL-1β to the hind paw skin [25]. More recently it has been shown that IL-1β can sensitize nociceptors by increasing the synthesis of substance P (a major nociceptive and inflammatory mediator) as well as the receptors that control its release [26]. In contrast, in inflamed tissue IL-1β has potent antinociceptive effects – an effect that has been attributed to IL-1β stimulation of endogenous opioid release from immune cells [27]. Recently, TNFα acting along the nerve trunk has been shown to elicit activity in nociceptive primary afferent fibres [28]. When injected into the peripheral receptive field, TNFα sensitizes receptors as well as eliciting discharge in afferent fibres [28]. There is also evidence that specific cytokines, e.g. TNFα and IL-6, play a role in the development of neuropathic pain behaviors [29, 30].

The complexity of mammalian nervous and immune systems makes detailed cellular analyses of immune mediated modulation of nociceptive function a challenging prospect. A useful approach is to develop simpler models that share fundamental mechanisms with mammalian systems. In this regard, molluscs and *Aplysia* in particular, represent unique model systems because they have relatively simple, well characterized nervous systems and furthermore, they share with mammals basic cellular defensive responses to non-self or wounded-self, i.e., the directed migration and accumulation of defense cells around foreign agents or at injured sites.

The molluscan cellular defence system

All invertebrates are endowed with remarkably effective internal defense systems that respond to injury and recognize and destroy foreign microbes that enter the body (reviewed in [31, 32]). Although molluscs lack an antibody-based immune system, some degree of specificity is conferred on the molluscan internal defense system by the presence of lectin-protein complexes that have the ability to opsonize and agglutinate non-self material [33, 34]. It is interesting that vertebrates have retained a family of non-immunoglobulin, lectin-like molecules (the pentraxins) of which C-reactive protein is an example [35]. The principal line of molluscan cellular defense is phagocytosis or encapsulation [36]. The hemocyte (also referred to as the amebocyte, leucocyte or immunocyte) which wanders freely in blood (hemolymph) and through loose connective tissue is the principal phagocytic cell. Although molluscs are protostome animals, not on a line of evolution leading directly to the vertebrates (Fig. 1), phagocytosis represents such a primitive mechanism that it would not be surprising if this capability evolved phylogenetically through common ancestors. Indeed, many similarities between molluscan hemocytes and phagocytic cells of the myeloid lineage (granulocytes and monocytes) have been demonstrated. For example, both molluscan hemocytes and mammalian macrophages use phagocytosis incorporating the release of highly reactive oxygen metabolites (e.g. hydrogen per-oxide, superoxide) and degradative enzymes (e.g. lysozyme, β-glucuronidase) as one of their defense strategies [37–40]. Nitric oxide, a macrophage bacteriocidal factor has recently been identified in molluscan hemocytes [41].

More recently, cells with a close structural and functional relationship to cellular defense cells have been identified in neural tissues of several invertebrate species including the leech [42, 43], the cockroach [44] and several different molluscs [45]. These structural and functional commonalities parallel those between vertebrate macrophages and microglia, thus these invertebrate cells have been compared to vertebrate microglia. A characteristic feature of microglia is their rapid activation in response to a variety of central nervous system (CNS) insults including injury, inflammation, neurodegeneration, infection and tumors [46]. In the leech, microglia move rapidly to nerve lesions in the CNS [47] and recent findings implicate these cells in regenerative processes following injury [48]. An understanding of the relationship between these invertebrate microglial-like cells and the nervous system could yield important information regarding the influence of microglia on neuronal functioning following injury in mammalian systems.

Invertebrate cytokines

As in vertebrate systems, cytokine-like factors appear to control many aspects of host defense responses in invertebrates. Even the most primitive invertebrates possess cytokine-like molecules. For example, there appears to be a structural and functional relationship between vertebrate IL-2 and a protozoan pheromone (Er-1) [49], and human IL-1β is an effective competitor of pheromone-receptor binding. Detectable levels of immunoreactive IL-1 and TNF are present in the hemolymph of a variety of molluscs including *Aplysia* [50, 51]. Preliminary analyses of cell lysate preparations support the notion that the hemocytes are the source of the cytokines detected in *Aplysia* hemolymph (A.L. Clatworthy and T.K. Hughes, unpublished observations).

Biochemical characterization of IL-1-like molecules from a number of deuterostome and protostome invertebrate species has revealed fundamental similarities in structure with vertebrate IL-1 [52, 53]. Furthermore, invertebrate IL-1 shares many biological activities with vertebrate IL-1. For example, in their native species, invertebrate IL-1-like molecules enhance cell proliferation, chemotaxis and phagocytic activity [54, 55]. Interestingly, media conditioned by hemocytes stimulated with zymosan significantly increased the proliferative and phagocytic activities of tunicate hemocytes – an effect that was associated with the release of tunicate IL-1 like factors by stimulated hemocytes [56]. More recently, an IL-6-like molecule has been identified in the mollusc *Mytilus edulis* [51] and in the coelomic fluid of the echinoderm *Asterias forbesi* [57]. Lipopolysaccharide (LPS) was shown to initiate release of the IL-6-like factor from coelomocytes (echinoderm cellular defense cells) [57]. These findings suggest that tunicate and echinoderm cytokine-like factors are expressed in response to selected antigenic stimuli.

IL-1-like factors isolated from an echinoderm (the starfish *Asterias forbesi*) and a variety of species of tunicate also show biological activity when assayed in vertebrate systems. For example, echinoderm and tunicate IL-1 stimulated thymocyte activity directly in the murine thymocyte proliferation assay and to a greater degree in the presence of submitogenic concentrations of concanavalin A [52, 58]. An antibody to human IL-1 was equally effective in inhibiting starfish IL-1-like factor and human IL-1 in the thymocyte assay. Echinoderm IL-1-like factors also enhance mammalian fibroblast proliferation and protein synthesis, stimulate release of prostaglandin E_2 and are cytotoxic to the human cell line A375 [58]. Both vertebrate and tunicate IL-1 produce an increase in vascular permeablity *in vivo* [53].

TNF-like and IL-2-like molecules have also been isolated from echinoderms and tunicates [53, 59]. Initial values for tunicate TNF Mr and pI of approximately 40–50,000 and 4, respectively, are comparable to mammalian TNF. Furthermore, invertebrate TNF is active in the murine L 929 fibroblast ctyotoxicity assay [58]. The ability of invertebrate cytokine-like molecules to have activity in vertebrate systems suggests that there is conservation of the three dimensional structure necessary for interaction with vertebrate cytokine receptors. However, the extent of homology shared between vertebrate and invertebrate cytokine-like molecules awaits more definitive analysis e.g. isolation and sequencing the cDNA clones encoding the cytokines.

Neural-immune interactions in *Aplysia*

Profound long-lasting increases in nociceptive sensory soma excitability and synaptic transmission can be produced in *Aplysia* following injury of peripheral nerves containing sensory axons ([20, 21], see also above). At least some of the signals are generated at the site of injury and transported to the soma via slow retrograde axonal transport [22]. One potential source of signals is factors released from the numerous hemocytes that are attracted to the injury site on the nerve (Fig. 4). In support of this idea, cytokines that have been localized to the hemocytes of a number of invertebrate species have been shown to have neuromodulatory actions in several molluscan species. For example, IL-1β and TNFα modulate ionic channels in the soma of identified neurons of the molluscs *Aplysia* and *Helix* [60–62].

To begin to test the hypothesis that hemocytes can influence sensory functioning, Clatworthy and colleagues examined whether an accumulation of hemocytes close to peripheral nerves can influence the excitability of sensory neurons having axons in those nerves [63]. A strip of cotton wrapped loosely around pedal nerves containing sensory axons served as the stimulus to activate the cellular defense system

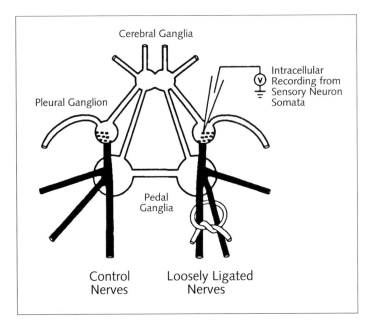

Figure 5
Preparation used to examine immune-mediated modulation of sensory excitability in Aplysia. A unilateral foreign body was induced by loosely ligating pedal nerves with a strip of cotton at a distance of approximately 1 cm from the pedal ganglion. The excitability of VC sensory neuron cell bodies (indicated by dots) having axons in ligated nerves was tested between 1 and 30 days later and compared to the excitability of contralateral VC sensory neurons having axons in non-ligated nerves. Modified after [63].

and produce an accumulation of hemocytes close to the peripheral nerves (Fig. 5). Contralateral pedal nerves were not ligated. Loose ligation of peripheral nerves induced a foreign body reaction as evidenced by the accumulation of numerous hemocytes around the cotton ligature. Five to 30 days after ligation, the excitability of the soma of nociceptive sensory neurons having axons in ligated nerves was significantly increased compared to contralateral, control sensory neurons having axons in non-ligated nerves. Spike threshold and afterhyperpolarization (AHP) were reduced, and spike amplitude and duration were increased. Sensory neurons on the ligated side also fired more spikes in response to a standard 1 sec intracellular depolarizing pulse compared to control sensory neurons. The recorded increase in sensory excitability is qualitatively similar to that seen following axonal injury [20, 21]. However, both morphological and electrophysiological evidence indicated that axons in ligated nerves were undamaged and able to conduct action potentials. Thus the effects are unlikely to be accounted for by ligation-induced injury of sensory axons. Also, the increase in action potential amplitude recorded following loose ligation is not associated with injury-induced sensory plasticity. Furthermore, the latency to onset of sensory hyperexcitability following ligation was approximately five days. This contrasts with the shorter latency (2–3 days) of sensory plasticity induced by crushing pedal nerves at a similar distance from the sensory cell body. The increased latency might reflect the time required for a sufficient number of hemocytes to aggregate close to sensory axons to exert an effect. Thus, the sensory changes associated with implantation of a foreign body close to peripheral nerves may be mediated by factors released from hemocytes that are activated by the presence of a foreign agent.

More direct evidence of a neuromodulatory role for molluscan hemocytes comes from some recent *in vitro* experiments. Crush-induced sensory hyperexcitability similar to that seen following nerve crush in intact animals can be recorded *in vitro* [22]. Thus, in isolated pedal/pleural ganglia preparations, pedal nerve crush will produce a significant increase in the excitability of nociceptive sensory neurons having axons in crushed nerves compared to sensory neurons having axons in uncrushed nerves. Although qualitatively similar, one difference between injury-induced sensory hyperexcitability *in vitro* and *in vivo* is that injury-induced sensory hyperexcitability is more profound *in vivo* (Clatworthy, unpublished observations). The *in vitro* preparation lacks hemocytes (besides those potentially present in the neural tissue); therefore, an interesting possibiblty is that factors released from activated hemocytes at the injury site *in vivo* may act to enhance the expression of injury-induced sensory hyperexcitability. To directly test this hypothesis, a second *in vitro* preparation was developed. One set of pedal-pleural ganglia was incubated in culture medium to which hemocytes were added. The contralateral control ganglia were incubated in the absence of hemocytes [64]. The associated peripheral nerves containing the sensory axons were cut short on both control and experimental sides so that the expression of injury-induced sensory hyperexcitability would be evident within 24 h. The influence of hemocytes on the expression of injury-induced sensory plasticity was tested after 24 h. Histological analysis of cross sections just proximal to the cut ends of peripheral nerves incubated in the presence of hemocytes revealed that numerous hemocytes were attracted to the cut end of the nerve. In contrast, very few hemocytes were associated with the cut end of the nerve that was incubated in the absence of hemocytes.

Electrophysiological analysis revealed that the AHP recorded from sensory cells incubated in the presence of hemocytes was lower and the spike duration longer compared to the AHP and duration recorded from sensory cells incubated in the absence of hemocytes. In addition, sensory cells incubated in the presence of hemocytes fired more spikes in response to a standard one second depolarizing pulse at 2.5 x spike threshold than control cells. Although there was a tendency for sensory cells incubated in the presence of hemocytes to be more excitable than sensory cells incubated in the absence of hemocytes, these differences were not significant.

In vertebrate systems, the endotoxin, LPS acts as a potent stimulator of monocytes/macrophages. It has been shown that the hemocytes of the mollusc *Mytilus edulis* respond to LPS (0.1 µg/ml) in a similar fashion to that observed in vertebrate systems – there is an increase in cell perimeter, flattening and an increase in mobility [65]. We were interested in determining whether the presence of LPS would enhance the expression of sensory hyperexcitability recorded in the previous experiments. Results from a series of preliminary experiments suggested that LPS alone could influence sensory excitability in *Aplysia*. To control for the effects of LPS on sensory excitability, the excitability of sensory cells incubated overnight in the presence of hemocytes and 0.1 µg/ml LPS was compared to the excitability of sensory cells incubated in 0.1 µg/ml LPS alone [64]. Sensory cells incubated in the presence of hemocytes and LPS were significantly more excitable than control cells. Spike AHP was significantly lower and the number of spikes evoked by a 1 sec depolarizing pulse at 1.25 x and 2.5 x spike threshold was significantly larger than that recorded from control sensory cells incubated in LPS alone (p < 0.05).

What are the potential hemocyte-derived factors mediating this enhancement of sensory excitability? Immunoreactive IL-1 and TNF have been detected in the hemolymph of *Aplysia* [50] and our studies suggest that the hemocytes are indeed the source of these cytokines. Preliminary studies demonstrating that IL-1 can enhance the expression of injury-induced sensory hyperexcitability *in vitro* suggest a role for IL-1 in this modulation of sensory function [50]. The stimulatory effects of LPS on *Mytilus* hemocytes were blocked by addition of antibodies specific for TNF and IL-1 which suggests that they are mediated by the release of IL-1 and TNF [65]. It is interesting to speculate that the addition of LPS to the incubation medium containing hemocytes enhanced the release of IL-1 (and perhaps other cytokine-like factors) which in turn potentiated the hemocyte-induced increase in sensory excitability recorded in the absence of LPS. In support of this hypothesis, preliminary studies suggest that in *Aplysia*, levels of circulating (ir) IL-1 and TNF are increased following administration of LPS *in vivo*.

Commonalities between invertebrate and vertebrate systems

When dealing with a simple system it is important to understand the relevance to more complex systems, i.e. will findings from the *Aplysia* model provide any useful information to groups as evolutionary divergent as molluscs and mammals which diverged very early in evolution when the deuterostomes separated from the protostomes (Fig. 1). The enhancement of responsiveness in *Aplysia* nociceptive sensory neurons following injury or the induction of a foreign body response is functionally similar to hyperalgesia (i.e. a heightened sensitivity to painful stimuli) in mammalian preparations. A mammalian model that has been used extensively to study neuropathic hyperalgesia that is associated with peripheral nerve injury involves loosely ligating the sciatic nerve in rats with chromic gut sutures [66]. Hyperalgesia is recorded from the paw on the ligated side within a few days. This rat model bears a striking resemblance to the model that has been used to study whether hemocytes can modulate nociceptive sensory functioning in *Aplysia* [63]. In both systems an increase in the responsiveness of nociceptive sensory neurons is produced following the induction of a cellular defense reaction close to peripheral nerves. Thus, in the rat model of neuropathic hyperalgesia, activated immune cells attracted to the chromic gut used to ligate the sciatic nerve may influence nociceptive processing.

The effect of manipulating the inflammatory response associated with the suture material used to ligate the nerve on the expression of hyperalgesia has been examined. Clatworthy and colleagues found that severely reducing the magnitude of the inflammatory reaction associated with chromic gut ligatures by treating the animals with the steroid dexamethasone significantly reduced the hyperalgesia recorded on the ligated side [67]. In contrast, enhancing the inflammatory response associated with cotton ligatures by soaking them in Freund's complete adjuvant prior to implantation significantly potentiated the hyperalgesic response associated with cotton sutures alone. These results suggest that inflammation in close proximity to the ligated sciatic nerve plays an important role in the development of hyperalgesia in this model of neuropathic pain.

Potential mediators of this hyperalgesic response include cytokines released from immune cells attracted to the chromic gut sutures. The expression of thermal hyperalgesia can be significantly reduced by administration of TNF-binding protein (an endogenous inhibitor of the cytokine TNFα) prior to the ligation [29]. This suggests that TNFα plays a role in the development of thermal hyperalgesia in this model of neuropathic pain and lends further support to the notion of an immune mediated modulation of nociceptive processing.

Conclusions

The overall goal of the studies in *Aplysia* is to generate results regarding fundamental mechanisms underlying neural-immune communication that can be used to formulate novel hypotheses in more complex systems. The feasibility of this approach is underscored by the fact that the recent studies showing an important role for the immune system in the development of hyperalgesia in a rat model of neuropathic pain [67] were designed on the basis of results from studies in *Aplysia* demonstrating an immune-mediated modulation of nociceptive sensory function [63].

Acknowledgements

I would like to thank Dr. E.T. Walters for helpful comments on this chapter and Amgen, Boulder Inc. for the donation of TNF binding protein.

References

1   Kavaliers M (1988) Evolutionary and comparative aspects of nociception. *Brain Res Bull* 21: 923–931

2   Walters ET (1994) Injury-related behavior and neuronal plasticity: an evolutionary perspective on sensitization, hyperalgesia and analgesia. *Int Rev Neurobiol* 36: 325–427

3   Kung C, Chang S-Y, Satow Y, Van Houten J, Hansma H (1975) Genetic dissection of behavior in paramecium. *Science* 188: 898–904

4   Corning WC, Kelly S (1973) Platyhelminths: the turbellarians. In: Corning WC, Dyal JA, Willows AOD (eds): *Invertebrate learning: Protozoans through annelids*. Plenum, New York, 171–224

5   Donaldson S, Mackie GO, Roberts A (1980) Preliminary observations on escape swimming and giant neurons in Aglantha digitale (Hydromedusae:Trachylina). *Can J Zool* 58: 549–552

6   Robson EA (1966) Swimming in actinaria. *Symp Zool Soc Lond* 16: 333–359

7   Ross DM (1968) Detachment of sea anemones by commensal hermit crabs and by mechanical and electrical stimulation. *Nature* 217: 380–381

8   Walters ET, Erickson MT (1986) Directional control and the functional organization of defensive responses in *Aplysia*. *J Comp Physiol* A 159: 339–351

9   Walters ET Byrne JH, Carew TJ, Kandel ER (1983) Mechanoafferent neurons innervating the tail of *Aplysia*. I. Response properties and synaptic connections. *J Neurophysiol* 50: 1522–1542

10   Clatworthy AL, Walters ET (1993) Rapid amplification and facilitation of mechanosensory discharge in *Aplysia* by noxious stimulation. *J Neurophysiol* 70: 1181–1194

11   Clatworthy AL, Walters ET (1993) Activity-dependent depression of mechanosensory discharge in *Aplysia*. *J Neurophysiol* 70: 1195–1209

12   Marcus EA, Nolen TG, Rankin CH, Carew TJ (1988) Behavioral dissociation of dishabituation, sensitization, and inhibition in *Aplysia*. *Science* 241: 210–212

13   Mackey SL, Glanzman DL, Small SA, Dyke AM, Kandel ER, Hawkins RD (1987) Tail shock produces inhibition as well as sensitization of the siphon-withdrawl reflex of *Aplysia* : possible behavioral role for presynaptic inhibition mediated by the peptide Phe-Met-Arg-Phe-NH2. *Proc Nat Acad Sci* 84: 8730–8734

14   Woolf CJ, Walters ET (1991) Common patterns of plasticity contributing to nociceptive sensitization in mammals and *Aplysia*. *Trends in Neurosci* 14: 74–78

15   Illich PA, Walters ET (1997) Mechanosensory neurons innervating *Aplysia* siphon encode noxious stimuli and display nociceptive sensitization. *J Neurosci* 17: 459–469

16   Price DD, Hull CD, Buchwald NA (1971) Intracellular responses of dorsal horn cells to cutaneous and sural nerve A and C fiber stimuli. *Exp Neurol* 33: 291–309

17   Woolf CJ, King AE (1987) Physiology and morphology of multireceptive neurons with c-afferent fibre inputs in the deep dorsal horn of the rat lumbar spinal cord. *J Neurophysiol* 58: 460–479

18   Walters ET (1987a) Site specific sensitization of defensive reflexes in *Aplysia*: a simple model of long-term hyperalgesia. *J Neurosci* 7 (2): 400–407

19   Walters ET (1987b) Multiple sensory neuronal correlates of site-specific sensitization in *Aplysia*. *J Neurosci* 7: 408–417

20   Walters ET, Alizadeh H, Castro GA (1991) Similar neuronal alterations induced by axonal injury and learning in *Aplysia*. *Science* 253: 797–799

21   Clatworthy AL, Walters ET (1994) Comparative analysis of hyperexcitability and synaptic facilitation induced by nerve injury in cerebral and pleural mechanosensory neurons of *Aplysia*. *J Exp Biol* 190: 217–238

22   Gunstream JD, Castro GA, Walters ET (1995) Retrograde transport of plasticity signals in *Aplysia* sensory neurons following axonal injury. *J Neurosci* 15: 439–448

23   Yaksh TL, Yamamoto T, Myers RR. (1992) Pharmacology of nerve compression-evoked hyperesthesia. In: Willis WD Jr (ed): *Hyperalgesia and allodynia*. Raven Press, New York, 245–258

24   Watkins LR, Wiertelak EP, Geohler LE, Smith KP, Martin D, Maier SF (1994) Characterization of cytokine-induced hyperalgesia. *Brain Res* 654: 15–26

25   Fukuoka H, Kawatani M, Hisamitsu T, Takeshige C (1994) Cutaneous hyperalgesia induced by peripheral injection of interleukin 1β in the rat. *Brain Res* 657: 133–140

26   Jeanjean AP, Moussaoui SM, Maloteaux, JM, Laduron PM (1995) Interleukin 1B induces long-term increase of axonally transported opiate receptors and substance P. *Neurosci* 68: 151–157

27   Stein C (1995) The control of pain in peripheral tissue by opioids. *N Engl J Med* 332: 1685–1690

28   Xiao WH, Wagner R, Myers RR, Sorkin LS (1996) TNFα in the peripheral receptive field or on the sciatic nerve trunk evokes activity in primary afferent fibres. *Soc Neurosci Abstr* 22: 1811

29   Illich PA, Martin D, Castro GA, Clatworthy AL (1997) TNF binding protein attenuates thermal hyperalgesia but not guarding behavior following loose ligation of rat sciatic nerve. *Soc Neurosci Abstr* 23: 166

30   DeLeo JA, Colburn RW, Nichols M, Malhotra A (1996) Interleukin-6-mediated hyperalgesia/allodynia and increased spinal IL-6 expression in a rat mononeuropathy model. *J Interferon Cytokine Res* 16: 695–700

31   Ratcliffe NA (1985) Invertebrate immunity – a primer for the non-specialist. *Immunol Lett* 10: 253–270

32   Clatworthy AL (1995) A simple systems approach to neural-immune communication. *Comp Biochem Physiol* 115(A): 1–10

33   Prowse RH, Tait NN (1969) In vitro phagocytosis by amebocytes from the hemolymph

of *Helix aspers* (Muller) I. Evidence for opsonic factors in the serum. *Immunol* 17: 437-443

34 Renwrantz L, Stahmer A (1983) Opsonizing effect of an isolated hemolymph agglutinin and demonstration of lectin-like recognition molecules at the surface of hemocytes from *Mytilus edulis. J Comp Physiol* 149: 535–546

35 Mold C, DuClos TW, Nakayama S, Edwards KM, Gerwurz T (1982) C-reactive protein reactivity with complement and effects on phagocytosis. *Ann NY Acad Sci* 389: 251–261

36 Tripp MR (1970) Defense mechanisms of mollusks. *J Reticuloendothel Soc* 7:173–182

37 Adema CM, van Deutekom-Mulder EC, van Der Knapp WPW, Meuleman EA, Sminia T (1991) Generation of oxygen radicals in hemocytes of the snail *Lymnaea stagnalis* in relation to the rate of phagocytosis. *Dev Comp Immunol* 15: 17–26

38 Leippe M, Renwrantz L (1988) Release of cytotoxic and agglutinating molecules by Mytilus hemocytes. *Dev Comp Immunol* 12: 297–308

39 Pipe RK (1990) Hydrolytic enzymes associated with the granular haemocytes of the marine mussel *Mytilus edulis. Histochem J* 22: 595–603

40 Pipe RK (1992) Generation of reactive oxygen metabolites by the haemocytes of the marine mussel *Mytilus edulis. Dev Comp Immunol* 16: 111–122

41 Ottaviani E, Paemen LR, Cadet P, Stefano GB (1993) Evidence for nitric oxide production and utilization as a bactericidal agent by invertebrate immunocytes. *Eur J Pharmacol* 248: 319–324

42 Coggeshall RE, Fawcett DW (1964) The fine structure of the central nervous system of the leech, *Hirudo medicinalis. J Neurophysiol* 27: 229–289

43 Morgese VJ, Elliott EJ, Muller KJ (1983) Microglial movement to sites of nerve lesion in the leech CNS. *Brain Res* 272: 166–170

44 Howes EA, Armett-Kibel C, Smith PJ (1993) A blood derived attachment factor enhances the *in vitro* growth of two glial cell types from the adult cockroach. *Glia* 8: 33–41

45 Sonetti D, Ottaviani E, Bianch F, Rodriguez M, Stefano ML, Scharrer B, Stefano GB (1994) Microglia in invertebrate ganglia. *Proc Natl Acad Sci* 91: 9180–9184

46 Barron KD (1995) The microglial cell. A historical review. *J Neurological Sci* 134: 57–68

47 McGlade-McCulloh E, Morrissey AM, Norona F, Muller KJ (1989) Individual microglia move rapidly and directly to nerve lesions in the leech central nervous system. *Proc Natl Acad Sci USA* 86: 1093–1097

48 Von Bernhardi R, Muller KJ (1995) Repair of the central nervous system: lessons from lesions in leeches. *J Neurobiol* 27: 353–366

49 Ortenzi C, Miceli C, Bradshaw RA, Luporini P (1990) Identification and initial characterization of an autocrine pheromone receptor in the protozoan ciliate *Euplotes raikovi. J Cell Biol* 111: 607–614

50 Clatworthy AL, Hughes TK, Budelmann BU, Castro GA, Walters ET (1994) Cytokines

may act as signals for the injury-induced hyperexcitability in nociceptive sensory neurons of *Aplysia*. *Soc Neurosci Abstr* 20: 557

51 Hughes TK, Smith EM, Leung, MK, Stefano GB (1992) Immunoreactive cytokines in *Mytilus edulis* nervous and immune interactions. *Acta Biologica Hungarica* 43: 269–273

52 Beck G, Habicht GS (1991) Primitive cytokines: harbingers of vertebrate defense. *Immunol Today* 12: 180

53 Beck G, Vasta GR, Marchalonis JJ, Habicht GS (1989) Characterization of interlukin-1 activity in tunicates. *Comp Bioch Physiol* 92 (B): 93–95

54 Beck G, O'Brien RF, Habicht GS, Stillman DL, Cooper EL, Raftos DA (1991) Invertebrate cytokines III: invertebrate interlukin-1 molecules stimulate phagocytosis by tunicate and echinoderm cells. *Cellular Immunol* 146: 284–299

55 Raftos DA, Cooper EL, Habicht GS, Beck G (1991) Tunicate cytokines: tunicate cell proliferation stimulated by an endogenous hemolymph factor. *Proc Natl Acad Sci USA* 88: 9518

56 Raftos DA, Cooper EL, Stillman DL, Habicht G, Beck G (1992) Invertebrate cytokines II: Release of interleukin-1-like molecules from tunicate hemocytes stimulated with zymosan. *Lymphokine Cytokine Res* 11: 235–240

57 Beck GB, Habicht GS (1996) Characterization of an IL-6-like molecule from an echinoderm (*Asterias forbesi*). *Cytokine* 8: 507–512

58 Beck G, O'Brien RF, Habicht GS (1989) Invertebrate cytokines: the phylogenetic emergence of interleukin-1. *Bioessays* 11: 62–67

59 Legac E, Vaugier GL, Bousquet F, Bajelan M, Leclerc M (1996) Primitive cytokines and cytokine receptors in invertebrates: the sea star *Asterias rubens* as a model of study. *Scand J Immunol* 44: 375–380

60 Sawada M, Hara N, Maeno T (1990) Extracellular tumor necrosis factor induces a decreased K conductance in an identified neuron of *Aplysia kurodai*. *Neurosci Letts* 115: 219–225

61 Sawada M, Hara N, Maeno T (1991a) Ionic mechanism of the outward current induced by extracellular injection of interleukin 1 onto identified neurons of *Aplysia*. *Brain Res* 545: 248–256

62 Szucs A, Stefano GB, Hughes TK, Rozsa KS, (1992) Modulation of voltage-activated ion currents on identified neurons of *Helix pomatia* by interleukin 1. *Cell Mol Neurobiol* 12: 429–438

63 Clatworthy AL, Castro GA, Budelmann BU, Walters ET (1994) Induction of a cellular defense reaction is accompanied by an increase in sensory neuron excitability in *Aplysia*. *J Neurosci* 14(5): 3263–3270

64 Clatworthy AL, Grose EF (1997) Immune cells release factors that modulate the excitability of nociceptive sensory neurons in *Aplysia*. *Soc Neurosci Abstr* 23: 166

65 Hughes TK, Smith EM, Barnett JA, Charles R, Stefano GB (1991) LPS stimulated invertebrate hemocytes: a role for immunoreactive TNF and IL-1. *Dev Comp Immunol* 15: 117–122

66 Bennett GJ, Xie Y (1988) A peripheral mononeuropathy in rat that produces disorders of pain sensation like those seen in man. *Pain* 33: 87–107

67 Clatworthy AL, Illich PA, Castro GA, Walters ET (1995) Role of periaxonal inflammation in the development of thermal hyperalgesia and guarding behavior in a rat model of neuropathic pain. *Neurosci Letts* 184: 5–8

Illness-induced hyperalgesia: Mediators, mechanisms and implications

Linda R. Watkins and Steven F. Maier

Department of Psychology, University of Colorado at Boulder, Boulder, CO 80309-0345, USA

Introduction

The focus of this chapter will be different from the others in this book as it takes a more holistic view of the organism. Such a view examines hyperalgesia from an adaptive perspective and makes the argument that exaggeration of pain is a natural and normal consequence of immune activation. During illness, infection, and injury, activated immune cells release substances that signal the brain, triggering a constellation of coordinated responses designed to enhance survival (for review, see Ref [1, 2]). Hyperalgesia will be argued to be simply one component of this brain-mediated illness response. There has been increasing recognition that the immune system is involved in the regulation of many diverse phenomena to which it has not previously thought to be relevant [2], and here we will argue that pain is such a phenomenon.

This chapter is organized into three sections. The first provides a brief overview of the basic immunology on which the rest of the chapter is based. In this first section, immune responses to infection and inflammation are described and the concept of the illness response is developed. The second section develops the arguments for hyperalgesia being part of this coordinated illness response and provides examples of the mechanisms that mediate these hyperalgesic states. The last section is highly speculative, as it attempts to describe potential implications of this work for basic and clinical pain research, as well as potential implications for the management of clinical pain.

Infection, inflammation and the illness response

How does the immune system respond to infection?

To understand the natural involvement of pain in the organism's response to immune activation, it is first necessary to understand a few basics about the functioning of the immune system. In terms of pain, the most relevant situations are infection and inflammation. These will be discussed in turn.

Infection occurs when cells of the immune system detect the presence of foreign cells (bacteria, yeast, viruses, etc.) or other "non-self" entities (tumors, endotoxin, senescent red blood cells, damaged cells, etc.). This detection triggers the activation of immune responses designed to eliminate the danger to the host by destruction and elimination of the "non-self" invaders. The ensuing immune responses are classically divided into two types, the first termed non-specific (or innate) immunity and the other termed specific (or acquired or adaptive) immunity [3].

Specific immunity will only be mentioned in passing here, as no clear evidence exists that it *per se* modulates pain, other than its involvement in initiating a generalized inflammatory response (see below). The specific immune response requires that immune cells identify the invader (the virus that produces measles versus the one that produces mumps, for example). This identification process, in turn, triggers a complex cascade of events requiring a variety of immune cell types. The end result of this process is the induction of effector mechanisms that can attack the invader and/or help in its elimination, such as the generation of antibodies (immunoglobulins) that are specific to the invader [3].

In contrast, the non-specific immune response is a very general, broad-spectrum response to anything deemed "non-self". Some forms of the innate immune response are preventative. The integrity of healthy skin, tears that wash bacteria from the eye, and acid in the stomach to kill microbes are common examples. Other forms of the innate immune response come into play when an invader successfully penetrates into the body. Even when invasion occurs, there is no need to recognize whether the invader is a polio virus versus an *E. coli* bacterium; that they are "non-self" is sufficient for triggering this generalized immune response [3].

The most common response to invasion is engulfment and digestion of the invaders by specialized phagocytic immune cells. There are many varieties of phagocytes, with the types perhaps most relevant to pain being neutrophils and macrophages (which migrate into various body tissues as well as the central nervous system), Kupffer cells (which perform surveillance for invaders in blood and lymph as these fluids pass through the liver), synovial A cells (in joints), and microglia (in the brain and spinal cord). All of these phagocytes, upon engulfing or contacting invaders, produce and release a series of proteins, one class of which are the proinflammatory cytokines. "Pro-inflammatory" refers to the fact that they trigger and enhance the inflammatory response (see below). Such cytokines include tumor necrosis factor (TNF), interleukin(IL)-1, IL-6, and IL-8 [3–5].

How does inflammation occur?

Both the specific and non-specific immune responses are involved in causing inflammation. Inflammation is a local response to tissue injury, infection, or irritants. In the case of bacteria invading through a skin cut, for example, inflammation limits bacterial spread, and kills and removes the bacteria through engulfment and digestion by phagocytes such as macrophages and neutrophils. Inflammation also initiates general tissue repair processes, involving proliferation of connective tissue, production of elastins and collagen, etc. [3].

As mentioned above, the release of proinflammatory cytokines is involved in the initiation and maintenance of inflammation. These substances produce inflammation by altering the capillaries in a manner which allows immune cells to pass into the inflamed tissue, by attracting immune cells to this site, and by activating the immune cells once they are at the site. The sources of the proinflammatory cytokines are diverse, including phagocytes as mentioned previously, but also including mast cells, fibroblasts, joint synoviocytes, keratinocytes in skin, endothelial cells of blood vessels, adrenal medulla chromaffin cells, gastrointestinal tract, bladder epithelial cells, etc. [3].

In addition, the inflammatory response involves at least four additional components, namely the complement system, kinin forming systems, fibrinolytic systems, and clotting factors. Together these act to increase fluid and cell entry into the inflammatory site via nitric oxide production, attract and activate immune cells, etc. [3].

Several points should be emphasized. First, there is strong positive feedback at every step of the inflammatory process. As one simple example, the production of IL-1 drives further production of more IL-1. Second, dramatic synergisms are the norm. For example, TNF and IL-1 can dramatically enhance each other's actions. Third, there are many fail-safes built into the immune response such that any end-point can be reached by multiple cell types and by multiple mechanisms.

The illness response – general considerations

A characteristic set of behavioral and physiological responses in humans and animals often follows immune activation by inflammation, injury, or infection. This constellation of changes has been called "illness" or "sickness" and includes fever, increased sleep (especially increased slow-wave sleep), decreased activity, decreased social interaction, decreased eating and drinking, decreased digestion, rapid formation of taste aversions to novel foods, release of adrenal corticosteroids, release of sympathetic catecholamines, and altered brain monoamine activity [1, 2, 6]. As we will show below, recent work from our laboratory and others strongly supports the idea that lowering of pain thresholds and exaggerated pain responses (hyperalgesia) are also aspects of this illness response [7].

The argument for why this particular constellation of illness responses occurs centers on the survival value of fever [6]. Fever is a highly adaptive response because raised body temperature inhibits bacterial and viral replication, enhances immune cell proliferation, activates enzymes that destroy invaders, etc. Indeed, it has been reported that decreasing fever can decrease survival [8, 9]. However, fever is not created without cost. Fever requires tremendous energy expenditure, as does proliferation of immune cells and tissue repair processes. However, energy must be generated to maintain these processes. It has been noted that the various aspects of the illness response can be viewed as behavioral and physiological mechanisms for saving and creating energy [6, 10]. The hormonal changes, for example, serve to release energy from body stores. Behavioral changes, such as increased sleep and decreased foraging for food, conserve energy. Similarly, hyperalgesia can be argued to discourage unnecessary activity and to enhance recuperation, thus conserving energy.

Inflammation, injury, and infection cause the illness constellation to occur by signaling the brain through the release of proinflammatory cytokines, especially TNF, IL-1 and IL-6 [1, 11]. Peripheral administration of these cytokines can create the entire illness response. Furthermore, infection models (such as administering lipopolysaccharide [LPS], the cell wall of Gram-negative bacteria associated with endotoxin) produce the illness response by inducing the release of proinflammatory cytokines, since the illness response can be attenuated simply by blocking the action of these cytokines with receptor antagonists or antisera [1, 11, 12]. Indeed, a variety of procedures commonly used in pain research to create exaggerated pain result in both the release of proinflammatory cytokines and illness responses. Such procedures include those that use killed bacteria (a key component of complete Freund's adjuvant), turpentine, zymosan (yeast cell walls), carrageenan (seaweed extract), tissue damage, and nerve damage [7, 13].

Once proinflammatory cytokines are released in the periphery, illness responses are produced as a result of signals reaching specific centers in the brain. This must be the case because fever, increases in sleep, decreases in social interaction, etc. are all organized and mediated by the brain. Brain lesions and centrally-administered drugs can block illness responses produced by peripheral infection or peripheral cytokine administration [12]. Peripherally-administered proinflammatory cytokines and LPS increase neural activity, alter neurotransmitter content, and activate protooncogenes (for example, activation of the immediate-early gene cFos) in discrete brain regions mediating illness responses [14–18].

Involvement of cytokines in the central nervous system

Signaling to the brain from proinflammatory cytokines released in the periphery during infection, inflammation, and injury has been termed "immune-to-brain communication". Early hypotheses of how such signaling occurs focused on the large, lipophobic proinflammatory cytokines reaching the brain via the bloodstream and then somehow crossing over into the central nervous system to create brain-mediated illness responses [1]. This possibility initially seemed attractive, especially since it was known that illness responses could be elicited not just by peripheral administration of IL-1 or LPS, but also by intracerebroventricular injection of these same substances [1, 12]. Furthermore, brain-mediated illness responses produced as a result of peripheral administration of IL-1 or LPS could be blocked by intracerebroventricular administration of IL-1 receptor antagonist, implying that critical cytokine receptors for creating illness responses were in fact within the brain itself [1, 12]. Such data appeared to imply that illness responses were actually produced by the direct action of proinflammatory cytokines in the central nervous system, rather than by action in the periphery.

These early hypotheses were only partially correct and there is dispute concerning the degree to which illness responses are actually created by blood-borne cytokines crossing the blood-brain barrier (see below). It is now clear that proinflammatory cytokines produced by infection, inflammation, and/or injury itself can activate certain peripheral nerves, with vagal sensory afferent nerves being most directly relevant to the present discussion. Once activated by proinflammatory cytokines, these peripheral nerves communicate with the brain and cause the release/synthesis of proinflammatory cytokines from cells (glia and perhaps neurons) within the central nervous system itself [19–21]. The cytokines released in the central nervous system, in response to peripheral nerve activation by peripheral cytokines, ultimately create illness responses. In the discussion that follows, the exact same arguments will be made for the induction of exaggerated pain responses following peripheral infection, inflammation, and injury.

Hyperalgesia as an illness response

By the early 1990's it became evident that neuroimmunologists studying the illness response and pain researchers studying exaggerated pain states could benefit from each other's work. At this time, several similarities between illness responses and pain responses were becoming evident. First, both had been argued to be motivated behaviors. For a pain researcher, pain as a motivator is clear but illness may be less so. Examples that illness responses are motivated include the facts that sick animals will (a) work to gain access to hot environments which aid in the creation of fever [8], (b) actively bar-press to stop a moving treadmill so that they can remain sedentary [22], and (c) increase food hoarding (despite illness-induced lack of eating) during situations of restricted food access [23]. Second, the description of the chronic phase of pain by Wall [24] is strikingly similar to the illness response. Wall noted that after an injury is sustained the organism enters, after a delay (during which infection/inflammation is undoubtedly occurring in their example), the chronic stage of pain typified by decreased activity, lack of eating and drinking, increased sleep, decreased social interaction, and enhanced pain [24]. All of these responses, except pain, were considered part of the classic illness response constellation in the early 1990's. Pain, at this time, had never been examined by neuroimmunologists, so its role in the illness response had not yet been determined. Third, it was striking that every model used to study hyperalgesia in the pain research literature induces the release of proinflammatory cytokines [7, 13], a fact not yet widely appreciated by pain researchers. Such models include, but are not limited to, arthritis models (involving injection of bacteria); nerve injury and constriction models; peripheral injection of formalin, zymosan, carrageenan, and the like; gout models; inflammatory bowel models; inflammatory bladder models; and so forth [7, 13]. Taken together, we decided to test whether infection and cytokines by themselves, in the absence of the usual hyperalgesia-inducing conditions, produce hyperalgesia as well as other illness responses and, if so, whether they are mediated by common pathways.

Hyperalgesia from intraperitoneal illness-inducing agents

The best-validated non-pathogenic model in the psychological literature for inducing transient illness in rats is the injection of intraperitoneal (i.p.) lithium chloride, so we used lithium chloride in our initial studies. Indeed, i.p. lithium chloride produced marked hyperalgesia [25, 26], as measured by the tailflick test. Seeking a more naturalistic infection model, we tested i.p. LPS with the rationale that it would mimic the presence of bacteria. This, too, produced marked hyperalgesia on the tailflick test which could not be accounted for either by changes in tail temperature or by generalized exaggerated reflex responses to all somatosensory stimuli [25–27]. Additionally, i.p. LPS produced exaggerated response to diverse pain stimuli (such as subcutaneous formalin), indicating generality across pain measures [26]. Peripheral cytokines were implicated since (a) the hyperalgesias produced by i.p. lithium chloride and i.p. LPS were each abolished by i.p. administration of a peripherally restricted IL-1 receptor antagonist [25], (b) i.p. LPS hyperalgesia could also be blocked by i.p. administration of a peripherally restricted TNF functional antagonist (TNF binding protein) [28] and (b) i.p. IL-1 and i.p. TNF each produced hyperalgesia as well [25, 29].

While investigating the mechanisms underlying these phenomena, we discovered that cutting the vagus nerve blocked this LPS-induced, IL-1-mediated hyperalgesia, whereas cutting visceral afferents to the spinal cord did not [30]. Indeed, cutting the vagus nerve also blocked i.p. IL-1-induced hyperalgesia and i.p. TNF-induced hyperalgesia [28, 29]. These data suggested that, for hyperalgesia following the i.p. administration of immune-activating agents, at least, (a) immune-to-brain communication occurs via peripheral nerves rather than by blood-borne cytokines and (b) the sensory neural signals generated by these i.p. agents are first transmitted to the brain, specifically via vagal sensory afferent nerves. In support of these possibilities, we have found that both i.p. LPS and i.p. IL-1 increase immediate-early gene (cFos) expression in sensory vagal neurons and in neurons of the nucleus tractus solitarius, the principal site of termination of vagal sensory afferent nerves in the brain [2, 31–33]. Furthermore, IL-1 has been reported to increase the electrical activity of vagal sensory afferent nerves [34] and our own preliminary electrophysiological studies indicate that i.p. LPS also increases activity in sensory vagal fibers [33].

But does such hyperalgesia actually belong as part of the illness response constellation? If it does, one would expect that cutting the vagus would disrupt other illness responses as well. This is in fact true. To date, ten different laboratories, using three different species, have shown that cutting the vagus disrupts every illness response examined, including fever, decreased social interaction, decreased feeding, increased sleep, hormonal changes, alterations in brain neurotransmitters, development of taste aversions, etc. [2]. Basically, if the vagus is severed, all of the brain-mediated illness responses to i.p. LPS or i.p. cytokines are eliminated or markedly reduced! Importantly, the effect of cutting the vagus is specific for disrupting illness responses produced by peripheral cytokines and LPS [2].

Regarding the neurocircuitry of illness-induced hyperalgesia, the initial circuitry is shared with all components of the brain-mediated illness response constellation. One direct action of i.p. proinflammatory cytokines appears to be binding to vagus-associated structures called paraganglia [35]. These bodies are comprised of glomus cells which express (at least) specific binding sites for IL-1. Paraganglia are chemoreceptors which form afferent synapses with sensory vagal fibers [36, 37]. Intriguingly, we have demonstrated that these paraganglia and vagal nerve fibers are anatomically unique with regards to their close proximity to nerve-associated lymphoid cells (NALC) [33]. Immune cells constitutively juxtaposed to the paraganglia-vagus nerves very rapidly increase their expression of both IL-1 and TNF following i.p. LPS [33]. The presence of IL-1 (and likely other inflammatory and immune-derived mediators as well) then leads to sensory signals to the brain [33, 34], presumably through activation of paraganglia. As the medullary nucleus tractus solitarius and associated structures are the principal termination site of vagal afferent fibers in the brain [38], these are thought to be the "hub" for concerted signaling to each of the diverse central nervous system areas that are responsible for creating each of the individual illness responses. In the case of illness-induced hyperalgesia, we have shown, with cFos immunohistochemistry and brain lesion studies that hyperalgesia occurs through a nucleus tractus solitarius – nucleus raphe magnus – spinal cord circuit, the descending component running through the spinal cord dorsolateral funiculus [30, 39].

An intriguing aspect of this illness hyperalgesia is that it appears to access spinal mechanisms previously discovered by studies of hyperalgesia which were induced by nerve damage and pharmacological stimulation of the spinal cord. That is, illness-induced hyperalgesia is prevented by spinal administration of competitive and non-competitive N-methyl D-aspartate (NMDA) antagonists, substance P antagonists, nitric oxide (NO) synthesis inhibitors, etc. [40, 41]. Thus inflammatory events, whether they be due to nerve trauma or to infective agents, may ultimately tap into common spinal pathways.

45

Hyperalgesia from subcutaneous inflammatory agents

The research reviewed above suggests that infection in the periphery activates a centrifugal circuit that ultimately activates the NMDA-NO cascade in the spinal cord. We have argued that cytokines released by immune cells in response to infectious agents are critical in the initiation of the hyperalgesia cascade produced by infection. This would suggest that processes other than infection, that also stimulate the synthesis and release of proinflammatory cytokines, should also produce hyperalgesia. Inflammation is an obvious example. Using formalin injected s.c. into the dorsum of a single hindpaw, we found reliable hyperalgesia as measured by the tailflick test [42]. Several striking similarities were found between this inflammation-induced hyperalgesia and the illness hyperalgesia described above. First, like illness-induced hyperalgesia, s.c. formalin hyperalgesia was blocked both by nucleus raphe magnus (NRM) lesions and by spinal transection, implicating a brain-to-spinal cord pathway [42]. Second, at the level of the spinal cord, inflammation likewise produced hyperalgesia via an NMDA-NO cascade [42]. Third, both i.p. LPS and s.c. formalin produced glial activation in dorsal spinal cord, as evidenced by immunohistochemistry [43]. Such glial activation appeared crucial to the induction of both i.p. bacteria and s.c. formalin hyperalgesias since each were abolished by fluorocitrate (a glial metabolic inhibitor) and CNI-1493 (a glial synthesis inhibitor) [43, 44]. It is notable that another form of inflammation-induced hyperalgesia, that produced by s.c. zymosan, is also blocked by such procedures [45].

But how could glia be involved in pain? At this point we knew that i.p. LPS induced rapid increases in IL-1 protein in dorsal spinal cord [2, 46], most likely from glia. Assuming similarities would exist between illness- and inflammation-induced hyperalgesias, we chose to test the effects of intrathecal IL-1 receptor antagonist on s.c. formalin hyperalgesia. Spinal IL-1 receptor antagonist blocked s.c. formalin hyperalgesia [44]. Furthermore, intrathecal antisera to nerve growth factor, another substance produced and released by activated glia, also prevented s.c. formalin hyperalgesia [44]. Selectivity of effect was observed as other products of activated glia (complement-3, TNF) did not appear to be involved since blockade of their actions was without effect on s.c. formalin hyperalgesia [44].

The blockade of s.c. formalin induced hyperalgesia by spinal IL-1 receptor antagonist is consistent with the facts that: (a) glial IL-1 production increases following either peripheral inflammation [47, 48] or exposure of glia to substance P [49–51], (b) neurons express receptors for IL-1 [52, 53], and (c) IL-1 receptor antagonist protects neurons from the excitotoxic effect of NMDA agonists [54]. Furthermore, IL-1 can activate glia to release nitric oxide and eicosanoids [55, 56], substances previously implicated in s.c. formalin hyperalgesia [57, 58]. Lastly, spinal administration of either LPS (which induces IL-1) or IL-1 (in combination with interferon gamma) produces hyperalgesia [45], likely through IL-1-mediated selective enhancement of nociceptive neuronal responses [59].

In addition, IL-1 stimulates exaggerated release of nerve growth factor from astrocytes [60, 61]. This is notable since we have shown that spinal administration of antiserum directed against nerve growth factor also blocked s.c. formalin hyperalgesia [44]. Glutamate [62], TNF [63], and LPS [64] also stimulate astrocyte nerve growth factor and strong synergism between IL-1 and TNF has been reported in this regard [60]. Nerve growth factor released from glia could influence afferent pain transmission by binding to high affinity receptors expressed by calcitonin gene-related peptide (CGRP) and substance P afferent fibers [65, 66] which terminate almost exclusively within lamina I and outer lamina II [67]. Indeed, nerve growth factor is known to influence neurotransmitter content in these terminals [68].

It is noteworthy that s.c. formalin hyperalgesia is also blocked by spinal administration of antagonists directed against nitric oxide synthesis and against substance P, NMDA, and non-NMDA excitatory amino acid receptors [42, 58, 69–71]. This is in keeping with the spinal release of substance P, glutamate, and aspartate known to occur following s.c. formalin [72, 73]. Furthermore, s.c. formalin hyperalgesia has been reported to be blocked by spinal administration of cyclooxygenase inhibitors [57]. Although typically thought to reflect actions on nocisponsive neurons, all of these observations are actually also consistent with the idea that glia play a key role in mediating inflammatory-induced and illness-induced hyperalgesic states. That is, glia: (a) express immunohistochemically detectable activation markers in response to NMDA agonists [74]; (b) release nitric oxide and aspartate in response to glutamate and excitatory amino acid agonists [75–77]; (c) release arachidonic acid and cyclooxygenase products in response to glutamate or substance P [56, 78–80]; (d) cause NMDA-mediated increases in intracellular calcium in nearby neurons due to glial release of glutamate and various excitatory amino acids [77, 81–83]; and (e) further increase extracellular glutamate by modulating the glial glutamate transporter, reducing glutamate uptake, and reducing the activity of the glial glutamate degradative enzyme, glutamine synthetase [82, 84–86].

Hyperalgesia from intrathecal glial stimulators

The data reviewed above argues that peripheral illness-inducing agents and peripheral inflammatory agents ultimately produce hyperalgesia via activation of spinal cord glia. If spinal cord glia are indeed key elements in mediating peripherally-induced hyperalgesias, direct activation of spinal cord glia should also produce hyperalgesia. Spinal administration of substance P, excitatory amino acids, nitric oxide donors, etc. will certainly activate glia. Such procedures, however, do not further our understanding of the specific role of glia since any results would be confounded by direct, simultaneous activation of neurons. A procedure that directly stimulates only glia is needed.

One approach is to take advantage of the fact that microglia are embryological-ly derived from immune cells [3]. Indeed, they function in the central nervous sys-tem as phagocytes, reactive to "non-self" similar to macrophages in the periphery. In addition, microglia and astrocytes frequently form positive feedback circuits, wherein activation of microglia stimulate astrocyte activation, which further stimu-late microglia, and so forth. In support of the usefulness of such an approach, Meller et al. reported that immune-stimulatory bacterial cell walls produced hyper-algesia following injection over spinal cord [45].

We are currently pursuing this approach using spinal administration of gp120, an HIV coat glycoprotein which stimulates immune responses by glia. Our interest in this agent derives in part from its potential as a pure glial stimulator, as neurons are not thought to respond directly to gp120. In response to gp120, astrocytes and/or microglia have been reported to release a wide array of substances including IL-1 [87, 88], nitric oxide [88, 89], glutamate [90], cysteine (an agonist at the NMDA receptor) [89] and other excitatory amino acids [90], IL-6 and TNF [91]. We are also focused on gp120 because it is potentially relevant to AIDS-related pain syndromes, since HIV readily gains access to the spinal cord during the course of the disease and thus may exaggerate pain in these patients by direct glial activation. What we know to date is that gp120 dose-dependently produces prolonged thermal hyperalgesia and allodynia following spinal administration, unconfounded by spread to supraspinal sites, motor disturbances, or altered tail temperature [92]. This hyperalgesic action of gp120 is consistent with a glial receptor-mediated action since disruption of the secondary and tertiary structure of gp120 (required for recep-tor binding to microglia and astrocytes; see [93]) abolishes its hyperalgesic action [92]. Further, we have demonstrated that spinal administration of gp120 rapidly and dramatically increases dorsal spinal cord levels of IL-1 (K.T. Nguyen, S.F. Maier and L.R. Watkins, unpublished observations), supporting a potential role of glial IL-1 in creating this hyperalgesic state. Thus it may be that direct glial activation can indeed produce hyperalgesia by actions within the spinal cord dorsal horn.

Implications for pain research

The work reviewed in this chapter has a number of potential implications for basic and clinical pain research, as well as for the management of clinical pain.

For basic pain research using animal models, the implications are derived from five aspects of the work. First, the potential involvement of peripheral and/or cen-tral cytokines in various animal pain models needs to be appreciated. As noted pre-viously, many of the subcutaneous, intraperitoneal, peripheral nerve, and visceral irritant/inflammatory models induce the production and release of proinflammato-ry cytokines as well as other immune-derived factors. In addition to the clear hyper-algesic effects of proinflammatory cytokines after s.c. injection (see other chapters in this book), robust hyperalgesia is also seen following proinflammatory cytokine injection into rat knee joint [94] and even hyperalgesia subsequent to substance P injection into knee joint can be prevented by interleukin-1 receptor antagonist [95]. Beyond such direct effects, indirect effects can occur as well. For example, bacterial translocation out of the lumen of the intestine and into the abdomen can occur under a surprisingly wide range of conditions. As one example, bacterial translocation can occur in response to colonic inflammation. Thus, colitis pain models may reflect, in part, illness-induced hyperalgesic effects consequent to bacteria (i.e. the live version of LPS) entry into the peritoneal lymphatics and immune organs draining this region. Second, regarding visceral pain models, it should be noted that the vagus innervates viscera more broadly than earlier appreciated. The colon, uterus, lungs, bladder, and other visceral tissues have all now been documented as receiving vagal sensory afferents. Since the response properties of vagal afferent neurons are quite diverse, with only a subpopulation mediating cytokine-to-brain communication, it is not yet known whether vagal innervation of the various visceral organs contributes to immune-to-brain communication. This potential warrants consideration in the use of such pain models. Third, peripheral cytokines may lead to the production of central cytokines. That is, peripheral cytokines activate afferent sensory nerves, leading to activation of illness/inflammatory pathways in the central nervous system, which ultimately activate central glia (and possibly neurons) to release cytokines and other factors. Thus, immune-derived substances can be involved in the periphery, the brain, and/or the spinal cord. Fourth, inflammation and illness lead to hyperalgesia which, at least for the models we have studied, involves a brain-to-spinal cord pathway. Given that even s.c. formalin hyperalgesia involves a brain-to-spinal cord pathway, it should not be tacitly assumed that a pain model is mediated simply at the level of the spinal cord, independent of the brain, without direct testing of the assertion [96]. Lastly, the potential involvement of spinal (and likely brain) glia warrants further study in a variety of pain states. Once microglia or astrocytes are activated, they can co-stimulate each other in positive feedback loops, driving the release and accumulation of proinflammatory cytokines, other classical immune products, and a host of substances (nitric oxide, glutamate, excitatory amino acids, arachidonic acid products, etc.) that have been documented to be important in driving various hyperalgesic states. What has been conceived to be a purely neuronal plasticity circuit for exaggerated pain responses may well be critically dependent on glia, at least in some circumstances.

Regarding relevance to human pain, we can only speculate. At a very general level, the present perspective may provide a different view of pain, one in which hyperalgesia is simply one of a whole constellation of brain-mediated changes triggered as a unit in response to illness signals. Thus, peripheral proinflammatory cytokines may be involved in conditions in which enhanced pain occurs concordantly with other aspects of the illness response (increased sleep, decreased eating, decreased social interactions, etc.). Immune-to-brain communication, in which activated immune cells inform the brain that infection, inflammation, and/or injury are occurring in the body is in keeping with the growing recognition that the immune system may function as a diffuse sensory system providing the brain with key information from the periphery. Indeed, spinal mechanisms for producing hyperalgesia could be argued to have evolved to subserve illness-induced hyperalgesia to support such recuperative responses.

In addition, the work reviewed here shows that illness-induced and inflammation-induced hyperalgesias can be controlled by three non-traditional methods. First, hyperalgesia induced by intraperitoneal injection of illness agents was blocked by complete subdiaphragmatic vagotomy. Blockage of illness-induced hyperalgesia by such a procedure is obviously not suggested as a means of pain control for humans. However, a point worth noting is that the vagal input to the brain that drives the hyperalgesic state is not the same nerve from which hyperalgesia appears to arise. In our studies, the nerves from which hyperalgesia appears to arise (based on the exaggerated pain response by the animal) were nerves from the tail that are responsive to the radiant heat of the tailflick test and the nerves from the hindleg carrying s.c. formalin pain. Thus the nerves creating hyperalgesia may be quite distinct (and quite distant) from the pain complaint. This has potential implications for a host of human situations in which activation of sensory vagal nerves may occur. These not only include the wide range of medical problems involving elevation of visceral and/or systemic proinflammatory immune products, but also possibly more subtle situations, such as viral infection/re-activation in the nodose ganglia containing the cell bodies of vagal sensory neurons. Herpes simplex virus, as one example, can harbor in both human [97] and mouse [98] nodose ganglia.

Second, hyperalgesia was prevented by blocking products of activated immune cells. Peripherally, such products include IL-1 and TNF. It is unlikely that these are the only substances leading to activation of illness-inducing vagal sensory afferent nerves. Peripheral actions of IL-1 and TNF lead to vagal transmission of illness signals to the brain, eliciting hyperalgesia along with the rest of the illness response. Hyperalgesia may be mediated in part by cytokines created and released in the central nervous system in response to afferent signals initiated by peripheral infection/inflammation. Thus cytokines can be involved simultaneously in the body, in the brain and/or in the spinal cord.

Third, hyperalgesia was controlled by inhibiting glial function using two drugs with very different mechanisms of action, and by inhibition of products of glial activation. This suggests that targeting spinal microglia and astrocytes (especially targeting their release of specific excitatory substances) may be an avenue worth exploring. This target may be important not only for pain of peripheral origin, but pain of central origin as well. Central nervous system infection, inflammation, and damage activate microglia and astrocytes, and release of their activation products would be expected to create and/or exaggerate pain if this release occurs near pain pathways. As an example, HIV and herpes viruses both activate glia. They could potentially exaggerate pain via release of immune and glial products at multiple sites: via their infection in peripheral tissues, via their infection of dorsal root ganglia, as well as via their infection of spinal cord. A centrally-driven component to virally-created pain states is clearly a concept worth further consideration.

Acknowledgments

This work was supported by NIH grants MH55283, MH45045, and RSA MH00314.

References

1   Watkins LR, Maier SF, Goehler LE (1995) Cytokine-to-brain communication: a review and analysis of alternative mechanisms. *Life Sci* 57: 1011–26
2   Maier SF, Watkins LR (1997) Cytokines for psychologists: implications of bi-directional immune-to-brain communication for understanding behavior, mood, and cognition. *Psych Rev* 105: 83–107
3   Kuby J (1992) *Immunology*. W. H. Freeman & Co., New York
4   Nathan CF (1987) Secretory products of macrophages. *J Clin Invest* 79: 319–326
5   Decker K (1990) Biologically active products of stimulated liver macrophages (Kupffer cells). *Eur J Biochem* 192: 245–261
6   Hart BL (1988) Biological basis of the behavior of sick animals. *Neurosci Biobehav Rev* 12: 123–137
7   Watkins LR, Maier SF, Goehler LE (1995) Immune activation: the role of pro-inflammatory cytokines in inflammation, illness responses and pathological pain states. *Pain* 63: 289–302
8   Kluger MJ (1991) Fever: role of pyrogens and cryogens. *Physiol Rev* 71: 93–127
9   Moltz H (1993) Fever: causes and consequences. *Neurosci Biobehav Rev* 17: 237–269
10 Maier SF, Watkins LR, Fleshner M (1994) Psychoneuroimmunology: the interface between behavior, brain, and immunity. *Amer Psych* 49: 1001–1018
11 Kent S, Bluthe R-M, Kelley KW, Dantzer R (1992) Sickness behavior as a new target for drug development. *Trends in Pharmacol Sci* 13: 24–28
12 Rothwell NJ, Luheshi G (1994) Pharmacology of interleukin-1 actions in the brain. *Adv Pharmacol* 25: 1–20
13 Walters ET (1994) Injury-related behavior and neuronal plasticity: an evolutionary perspetive on sensitization, hyperalgesia, and analgesia. *Int Rev Neurobiol* 36: 325–427
14 Dunn AJ (1993) Role of cytokines in infection-induced stress. *Ann NY Acad Sci* 697: 189–202
15 Dunn AJ (1988) Systemic interleukin-1 administration stimulates hypothalamic norepinephrine metabolism parallelling the increased plasma corticosterone. *Life Sci* 43: 429–435

16   Wan W, Wetmore L, Sorensen CM, Greenberg AH, Nance DM (1994) Neural and bio-chemical mediators of endotoxin and stress-induced c-fos expression in the rat brain. *Brain Res Bull* 34: 7–14

17   Ericsson A, Kovacs KJ, Sawchenko PE (1994) A functional anatomical analysis of central pathways subserving the effects of interleukin-1 on stress-related neuroendocrine neurons. *J Neurosci* 14: 897–913

18   Saphier D (1989) Neurophysiological and endocrine consequences of immune activity. *Psychoneuroendo* 14: 63–87

19   Ban E, Haour F, Lenstra R (1992) Brain interleukin1 gene expression induced by peripheral lipopolysaccharide administration. *Cytokine* 4: 48–54

20   Gatti S, Bartfai T (1993) Induction of tumor necrosis factor-a mRNA in the brain after peripheral endotoxin treatment: comparison with interleukin-1 family and interleukin-6. *Brain Res* 624: 291–294

21   Laye S, Bluthe R-M, Kent S, Combe C, Medina C, Parnet P, Kelley K, Dantzer R (1995) Subdiaphragmatic vagotomy blocks the induction of interleukin-1β mRNA in the brain of mice in response to peripherally administered lipopolysaccharide. *Am J Physiol* 268: R1327–R1331

22   Miller NE (1961) Some psychophysiological studies of motivation and of the behavioral effects of sickness. *Bull Brit Psych Soc* 17: 1–20

23   Aubert A, Kelley KW, Dantzer R (1997) Differential effect of lipopolysaccharide on food hoarding behavior and food consumption in rats. *Brain, Behavior & Immunity* 11: 229–238

24   Wall PD (1979) On the relation of injury to pain. The John J. Bonica lecture. *Pain* 6: 253–264

25   Maier SF, Wiertelak EP, Martin D, Watkins LR (1993) Interleukin-1 mediates behavioral hyperalgesia produced by lithium chloride and endotoxin. *Brain Res* 623: 321–324

26   Wiertelak EP, Smith KP, Furness L, Mooney-Heiberger K, Mayr T, Maier SF, Watkins LR (1994) Acute and conditioned hyperalgesic responses to illness. *Pain* 56: 227–234

27   Mason P (1993) Lipopolysaccharide induces fever and decreases tail flick latency in awake rats. *Neurosci Lett* 154: 134–136

28   Watkins LR, Wiertelak EP, Goehler LE, Smith KP, Martin D, Maier SF (1994) Characterization of cytokine-induced hyperalgesia. *Brain Res* 654: 15–26

29   Watkins LR, Goehler LE, Relton J, Brewer MT, Maier SF (1995) Mechanisms of tumor necrosis factor-alpha (TNF-alpha) hyperalgesia. *Brain Res* 692: 244–250

30   Watkins LR, Wiertelak EP, Goehler LE, Mooney-Heiberger K, Martinez J, Furness L, Smith KP, Maier SF (1994) Neurocircuitry of illness-induced hyperalgesia. *Brain Res* 639: 283–299

31   Goehler LE, Gaykema RPA, Tilders FJH, Maier SF, Watkins LR (1996) Endotoxin induces Fos immunoreactivity in rat vagal sensory ganglion cells. In: *International Society for Neuroimmunomodulation*. Washington, DC

32   Gaykema RPA, Goehler LE, McGorry MM, Milligan ED, Fleshner M, Tilders FJH, Maier SF, Watkins LR (1997) Subdiaphragmatic vagotomy inhibits fos expression in

brain and pituitary after intraperitoneal but not intravenous administration of endotoxin. *Proc Soc Neurosci* 23: 1514

33 Hammack SE, Nguyen KT, Hinde JL, Gaykema RPA, Goehler LE, Maier SF, Watkins LR (1998) Does IL-1beta activate the vagus nerve? LPS induces IL-1beta in the vagus nerve and intraperitoneal IL1beta injections increase firing rate in vagal afferents. In: *Psychoneuroimmunology Research Society meeting*. Bristol, England

34 Niijima A (1996) The afferent discharges from sensors for interleukin 1 beta in the hepatoportal system in the anesthetized rat. *J Auton Nerv Syst* 61: 287–291

35 Goehler LE, Relton JK, Dripps D, Kiechle R, Tartaglia N, Maier SF, Watkins LR (1997) Vagal paraganglia bind biotinylated interleukin-1 receptor antagonist (IL-1ra) in the rat: a possible mechanism for immune-to-brain communication. *Brain Res Bull* 43: 357–364

36 Morgan M, Pack RJ, Howe A (1976) Structure of cells and nerve endings in abdominal vagal paraganglia of the rat. *Cell Tiss Res* 169: 467–484

37 Berthoud H-R, Powley TL (1993) Characterization of vagal innervation to the rat celiac, suprarenal and mesenteric ganglia. *J Auto Nerv Sys* 42: 153–170

38 Ritter S, Ritter RC, Barnes CD (eds) (1992) *Neuroanatomy and physiology of abdominal vagal afferents*. CRC Press, Ann Arbor

39 Wiertelak EP, Roemer B, Maier SF, Watkins LR (1997) Comparison of the effects of nucleus tractus solitarius and ventral medulla lesions on illness-induced and subcutaneous formalin-induced hyperalgesias. *Brain Res* 748: 143–150

40 Wiertelak EP, Furness LE, Watkins LR, Maier SF (1994) Illness-induced hyperalgesia is mediated by a spinal NMDA-nitric oxide cascade. *Brain Res* 664: 9–16

41 Watkins LR, Wiertelak EP, Furness LE, Maier SF (1994) Illness-induced hyperalgesia is mediated by spinal neuropeptides and excitatory amino acids. *Brain Res* 664: 17–24

42 Wiertelak EP, Furness LE, Horan R, Martinez J, Maier SF, Watkins LR (1994) Subcutaneous formalin produces centrifugal hyperalgesia at a non-injected site via the NMDA-nitric oxide cascade. *Brain Res* 649: 19–26

43 Watkins LR, Deak T, Silbert L, Martinez J, Goehler L, Relton J, Martin D, Maier SF (1995) Evidence for involvement of spinal cord glia in diverse models of hyperalgesia. *Proc Soc Neurosci* 21: 897

44 Watkins LR, Martin D, Ulrich P, Tracey KJ, Maier SF (1997) Evidence for the involvement of spinal cord glia in subcutaneous formalin induced hyperalgesia in the rat. *Pain* 71: 225–235.

45 Meller ST, Dyskstra C, Grzybycki D, Murphy S, Gebhart GF (1994) The possible role of glia in nociceptive processing and hyperalgesia in the spinal cord of the rat. *Neuropharmacol* 33: 1471–1478

46 Nguyen KT, Deak T, Owens SM, Fleshner M, Watkins LR, Maier SF (1997) Effects of LPS and acute stress on rat brain interleukin-1beta. *Proc Soc Neurosci* 23: 715

47 Buttini M, Boddeke H (1995) Peripheral lipopolysaccharide stimulation induces interleukin-1b messenger RNA in rat brain microglial cells. *Neurosci* 65: 523–530

48 VanDam AM, Brouns M, Louisse S, Berkenbosch F (1992) Appearance of interluekin-1

in macrophages and in ramified microglia in the brain of endotoxin-treated rats: a pathway for the induction of non-specific symptoms of sickness? *Brain Res* 588: 291–298

49 Martin FC, Charles AC, Sanderson MJ, Merrill JE (1992) Substance P stimulates IL-1 production by astrocytes via intracellular calcium. *Brain Res* 599: 13–18

50 Martin FC, Anton PA, Gornbein JA, Shanahan F, Merrill JE (1993) Production of interleukin-1 by microglia in response to substance P: role for a non-classical NK-1 receptor. *J Neuroimmunol* 42: 53–60

51 Luber-Narod J, Kage R, Leeman SE (1994) Substance P enhances the secretion of tumor necrosis factor-alpha from neuroglial cells stimulated with lipopolysaccharide. *J Immunol* 152: 819–824

52 Ericsson A, Liu C, Hart RP, Sawchenko PE (1995) Type 1 interleukin-1 receptor in the rat brain: distribution, regulation, and relationship to sites of IL-1-induced cellular activation. *J Comp Neurol* 361: 681–698

53 Takao T, Hashimoto K, DeSouza EB (1995) Interleukin-1 receptors in the brain-endocrine-immune axis. *Ann NY Acad Sci* 771: 372–385

54 Relton JK, Rothwell NJ (1992) Interleukin-1 receptor antagonist inhibits ischaemic and excitotoxic neuronal damage in the rat. *Brain Res* Bull 29: 243–246

55 Hewett SJ, Corbett JA, McDaniel ML, Choi DW (1993) Interferon-gamma and interleukin-1beta induce nitric oxide formation from primary mouse astrocytes. *Neurosci Lett* 164: 229–232

56 Marriott D, Wilkin GP, Coote PR, Wood JN (1991) Eicosanoid synthesis by spinal cord astrocytes is evoked by substance P; possible implications for nociception and pain. *Adv Prostaglandin Thromboxane Leukot Res* 21B: 739–741

57 Malmberg AB, Rafferty MF, Yaksh TL (1994) Antinociceptive effect of spinally delivered prostaglandin E receptor antagonists in the formalin test on the rat. *Neurosci Lett* 173: 193–196

58 Yamamoto T, Shimoyama N, Mizuguchi T (1993) Nitric oxide synthase inhibitor blocks spinal sensitization induced by formalin injection into the rat paw. *Anesth Analg* 77: 886–890

59 Oka T, Aou S, Hori T (1994) Intracerebroventircula injection of interleukin-1 beta enhances nociceptive neuronal responses of the trigeminal nucleus caudalis in rats. *Brain Res* 656: 236–244

60 Gadient RA, Cron KC, Otten U (1990) Interleukin-1β and tumor necrosis factor-alpha synergistically stimulate nerve growth factor (NGF) release from cultured rat astrocytes. *Neurosci Lett* 117: 335–340

61 Carman-Krzan M, Vige X, Wise BC (1991) Regulation by interleukin-1 of nerve growth factor secretion and nerve growth factor mRNA expression in rat primary astroglial cultures. *J Neurochem* 56: 636–643

62 Pechan PA, Chowdhury K, Gerdes W, Seifert W (1993) Glutamate induces the growth factors NGF, bFGF, the receptor FGF-R1 and c-fos mRNA expression in rat astrocyte culture. *Neurosci Lett* 153: 111–114

63 Hattori A, Tanaka E, Murase K, Ishida N, Chatani Y, Tsujimoto M, Hayashi K, Kohno

M (1993) Tumor necrosis factor stimulates the synthesis and secretion of biologically actie nerve growth factor in non-neuronal cells. *J Biol Chem* 268: 2577–2582

64   Friedman WJ, Larkfors L, Ayer-LeLievre C, Ebendal T, Olson L, Persson H (1990) Regulation of beta-nerve growth factor expression by inflammatory mediators in hippocampal cultures. *J Neurosci Res* 27: 374–382

65   Averill S, McMahon SB, Clary DO, Reichardt LF, Preistley JV (1994) Immunocytochemical localisation of trkA receptors in chemically identified subgrouops of adult sensory neurones. *Eur J Neurosci* 1484–1494

66   Verge VM, Richardson PM, Benoit R, Riopelle RJ (1989) Histochemical characterization of sensory neurons with high-affinity receptors for nerve growth factor. *J Neurocytol* 18: 583–591

67   Yip HK, Johnson EM (1987) Nerve growth factor receptors in rat spinal cord: an autoradiographic and immunohistochemical study. *Neurosci* 22: 267–279

68   Verge VM, Richardson PM, Wiesenfeld-Hallin Z, Hokfelt T (1995) Differential influence of nerve growth factor on neuropeptide expression *in vivo*: a novel role in peptide suppression in adult sensory neurons. *J Neurosci* 15: 2081–2096

69   Coderre TJ, Melzack R (1992) The role of NMDA receptor-operated calcium channels in persistent nociception after formalin-induced tissue injury. *J Neurosci* 12: 3671–3675

70   Coderre TJ, Melzack R (1992) The contribution of excitatory amino acids to central sensitization and persistent nociception after formalin-induced tissue injury. *J Neurosci* 12: 3665–3670

71   Coderre TJ, Katz J, Vaccarino AL, Melzack R (1993) Contribution of central neuroplasticity to pathological pain: review of clinical and experimental evidence. *Pain* 52: 259–285

72   Skilling SR, Smullin DH, Beitz AJ, Larson AA (1988) Extracellular amino acid concentrations in the dorsal spinal cord of freely moving rats following veratridine and nociceptive stimulation. *J Neurochem* 51: 127–132

73   Smullin DH, Skilling SR, Larson AA (1990) Interactions between substance P, calcitonin gene-related peptide, taurine, and excitatory amino acids in the spinal cord. *Pain* 42: 93–101

74   Garrison CJ, Dougherty PM, Kajander KC, Carlton SM (1991) Staining of glial fibrillary acidic protein (GFAP) in lumbar spinal cord increases following a sciatic nerve constriction injury. *Brain Res* 565: 1–7

75   Agullo L, Baltrons MA, Garcia A (1995) Calcium-dependent nitric oxide formation in glial cells. *Brain Res* 686: 160–168

76   Simmons ML, Murphy S (1992) Induction of nitric oxide synthase in glial cells. *J Neurochem* 59: 897–905

77   McKenna MC, Sonnewald U, Huang X, Stevenson J, Zielke HR (1996) Exogenous glutamate concentration regulates the metabolic fate of glutamate in astrocytes. *J Neurochem* 66: 386–393

78   Stella N, Tence M, Glowinski J, Premont J (1994) Glutamate-evoked release of arachidonic acid from mouse brain astrocytes. *J Neurosci* 14: 568–75

79   Hartung H-P, Heininger K, Schafer B, Toyka KV (1988) Substance P and astrocytes: stimulation of the cyclooxygenase pathway of arachidonic acid metabolism. *FASEB J* 2: 48–51

80   Marriott DR, Wilkin G, Wood JN (1991) Substance P-induced release of prostaglandins from astrocytes: regional specialisation and correlation with phosphoinositol metabolism. *J Neurochem* 56: 259–265

81   Dutton G (1993) Astrocyte amino acids: evid)ence for release and possible interactions with neurons. In: Murphy S (ed): *Astrocytes: Pharmacology and function.* Academic Press, San Diego, 173–192

82   Muller CM (1992) A role for glial cells in activity-dependent central nervous plasticity? Review and hypothesis. *Internat Rev Neurobiol* 34: 215–281

83   Parpura V, Basarsky TA, Liu F, Jeftinija K, Jeftinija S, Haydon PG (1994) Glutamate-mediated astrocyte-neuron signalling. *Nature* 369: 744–747

84   Paini D, Frei K, Pfister HW, Fontana A (1993) Glutamate uptake by astrocytes is inhibited by reactive oxygen intermediates but not by other macrophage-derived molecules including cytokines, leukotrienes or platelet-activating factor. *J Neuroimmunol* 48: 153–156

85   Barbour B, Szatkowski M, Ingledew N, Attwell D (1989) Arachidonic acid induces a prolonged inhibition of glutamate uptake into glial cells. *Nature* 342: 918–920

86   McBean GJ, Doorty KB, Tipton KF, Kollegger H (1995) Alteration in the glial cell metabolism of glutamate by kainate and N-methyl-D-aspartate. *Toxicon* 33: 569–576

87   Merrill JE, Koyanagi Y, Zack J, Thomas L, Martin F, Chen IS (1992) Induction of interleukin-1 and tumor necrosis factor alpha in brain cultures by human immunodeficiency virus type 1. *J Virol* 66: 2217–2225

88   Koka P, He K, Zack JA, Kitchen S, Peacock W, Fried I, Tran T, Yashar SS, Merrill JE (1995) Human immunodeficiency virus 1 envelope proteins induce interleukin 1, tumor necrosis factor alpha, and nitric oxide in glial cultures derived from fetal, neonatal, and adult human brain. *J Exp Med* 182: 941–951

89   Lipton SA, Yeh M, Dreyer EB (1994) Update on current models of HIV-related neuronal injury: platelet-activating factor, arachidonic acid and nitric oxide. *Adv Neuroimmunol* 4: 181–8

90   Dreyer EB, Lipton SA (1995) The coat protein gp120 of HIV-1 inhibits astrocyte uptake of excitatory amino acids via macrophage arachidonic acid. *Eur J Neurosci* 7: 2502–2507

91   Clouse KA, Cosentino LM, Weih KA, Pyle SW, Ribbins PB, Hochstein HD, Natarajan V, Farrar WL (1991) The HIV-1 gp120 envelope protein has the intrinsic capacity to stimulate monokine secretion. *J Immunol* 147: 2892–2901

92   Milligan ED, Hinde JL, Maier SF, Watkins LR (1997) The HIV-1 coat protein, gp120, produces thermal hyperalgesia in rats. *Proc Soc Neurosci* 23: 1805

93   Sundar SK, Cierpial MA, Kamaraju LS, Long S, Hsieh S, Lorenz C, Aaron M, Ritchie JC, Weiss JM (1991) Human immunodeficiency virus glycoprotein (gp120) infused into

rat brain induces interleukin 1 to elevate pituitary-adrenal activity and decrease peripheral cellular immune responses. *Proc Natl Acad Sci* 88: 11246–11250

94 Davis, AJ, Perkins MN (1994) The involvement of bradykinin B1 and B2 receptor mechanisms in cytokine-induced mechanical hyperalgesia in the rat. *Brit J Pharmacol* 113: 63–68

95 Davis AJ, Perkins MN (1996) Substance P and capsaicin-induced mechanical hyperalgesia in the rat knee joint: the involvement of bradykinin B1 and B2 receptors. *Brit J Pharmacol* 118: 2206–2212

96 Watkins LR, Maier SF (1997) The case of the missing brain: arguments for a role of brain-to-spinal cord pathways in pain facilitation. *Behav Brain Sci* 20: 469

97 Gesser RM, Koo SC (1997) Latent herpes simplex virus type 1 gene expression in ganglia innervating the human gastrointestinal tract. *J Virol* 71: 4103–4106

98 Gesser RM, Valyi-Nagy T, Altschuler SM, Fraser NW (1994) Oral-oesophageal inoculation of mice with herpes simplex virus type I causes latent infection of the vagal sensory ganglia (nodose ganglia). *J Gen Virol* 75: 2379–2386

Hyperalgesia from subcutaneous cytokines

Stephen Poole[1], Fernando de Queiroz Cunha[2] and Sergio Henriques Ferreira[2]

[1]Division of Endocrinology, National Institute for Biological Standards and Control, Blanche Lane, South Mimms, Potters Bar, Herts EN6 3QG, UK; [2]Department of Pharmacology, Faculty of Medicine of Ribeirão Preto, University of São Paulo, Ribeirão Preto, Brazil

General concepts

Cytokines

Cytokines are proteins produced by cells in response to a variety of stimuli: they are released by their producer cells and act upon receptors on target cells. Cytokines may be produced by more than one cell type and in a number of tissues and may work in an autocrine, paracrine, or endocrine manner. All cytokines are small proteins (typically 5–30 kDa), some are glycoproteins, and some are synthesised as larger precursors which are cleaved to give the active molecule. As expected of agents that have a number of regulatory roles, cytokines are rarely produced at a constant rate but rather their production is induced (or suppressed) by specific stimuli to which the organism needs to respond. The lifetimes of cytokines are generally short and their destruction/clearance is usually a regulated process. Cytokines have essential roles in the control of cell proliferation, during embryonic development and in later life, and they are involved in regulating the immune response to foreign antigens on invading organisms. Essential processes such as cellular renewal and wound healing, the development of cellular and humoral immunity, and inflammatory responses all require participation of a range of cytokines. It is not surprising, therefore, that many diseases and conditions involving disruption of these processes are associated with altered regulation of cytokine production and action.

Interleukins and tumour necrosis factor

Interleukins act as inter-cellular signalling agents between leukocytes, hence their name. In fact, interleukins are produced by, and act upon, a variety of cell types, including monocytes, macrophages and lymphocytes. Some have been assigned numbers according to the chronology of their discovery, e.g. interleukin-1 (IL-1), while others have been named after a biological activity, e.g. tumour necrosis factor

(TNF). Cytokines that are believed to have major roles in inflammatory events are IL-1 (IL-1α and IL-1β, two separate gene-products), IL-6, IL-8 and TNFα [1].

Anti-inflammatory cytokines

An increasing number of cytokines have been shown to have activities which oppose or down-regulate inflammatory processes. Among these are the IL-1 receptor antagonist (IL-1ra), IL-4, IL-10, IL-12, IL-13 and transforming growth factor-β (TGFβ). These cytokines are believed to modulate immune and inflammatory events, allowing resolution of the inflammation and a return of the inflamed tissue to its normal state [1].

Nociceptive test

The first reports to suggest a role for cytokines in mediating inflammatory hyperalgesia appeared some ten years ago [2–4]. The model used in two of the first three publications [2, 4], and in many of the studies sited below, was a rat paw pressure test of mechanical hyperalgesia following injection of the cytokine into a hind-paw (intraplantar, i.pl.) [5]. A constant pressure of 20 mm Hg was applied to the hind-paws of rats and discontinued when they presented a typical freezing reaction (reaction time). This reaction was characterised by a reduction of escape movements: animals usually made several attempts to escape from the position imposed by the experimental situation. This activity was followed by alterations in respiratory frequency with the onset of a typical shivering reaction. The intensity of hyperalgesia was quantified as the variation in reaction time (delta reaction time) obtained by subtracting values measured after intraplantar (i.pl.) administration of a hyperalgesic agent from (control) reaction times, measured before injection of the hyperalgesic agent.

In the experiments described below, hyperalgesia was measured after injection of cytokines (human recombinant, h.r., unless indicated otherwise) and other hyperalgesic agents, each injected in into a hind paw (100 μl, intraplantar, i.pl.) in rats. Anti-hyperalgesic agents (inhibitors, antagonists, and antibodies) were injected (in 50 to 150 μl, i.pl., unless indicated otherwise) into paws to be injected with a hyperalgesic agent 30 min before the hyperalgesic agents (unless indicated otherwise). The doses of hyperalgesic agents were frequently the smallest doses that evoked maximum responses.

Sensitisation of the primary sensory neurone (PSN)

Sensitisation of the pain receptor is the common denominator of all types of pain which have an inflammatory element, that is 'inflammatory pain'. C-polymodal, high threshold receptors or receptors connected by fine myelinated fibres have long been associated with inflammatory hyperalgesia. More recently, a 'sleeping' pain receptor (nociceptor) associated with a small afferent fibre, has been described in deep visceral innervation (colon and bladder) and in joints [6]. Sleeping nociceptors cannot be activated in normal (healthy) tissues but are 'switched on' during inflammation. Clinically this functional up-regulation of pain receptors is referred to as hyperalgesia. In the hyperalgesic state, previously ineffective stimuli are painful.

There are two distinct groups of inflammatory mediators that affect PSNs: those which directly sensitise PSN and those which activate sensitised pain receptors. In the hyperalgesic state, previously ineffective stimuli cause 'overt pain' because they are now able to activate the sensitised nociceptors. Hyperalgesic agents that satisfy clinical and experimental criteria for directly-acting 'nociceptor sensitisers' are the products of arachidonic acid/cyclo-oxygenase, e.g. prostaglandins (PGs), and also the sympathomimetic amines.

The capacity of the PGs (PGE_2, PGI_2) to sensitise PSN has been studied extensively in man and in experimental animals using both behavioural and electrophysiological techniques [7–9].

Noradrenaline, dopamine and serotonin (5-hydroxytrytamine) have all been shown to functionally up-regulate nociceptors [10]. Consistent with this finding, depletion by guanethidine of peripheral sympthomimetic amines, treatment with adrenoceptor antagonists (beta-blockers) or with the dopamine (DA_1) antagonist SCH 23390 reduced responses to the hyperalgesic agent carrageenin. These antagonists also abolished hyperalgesic responses (in rat paws) to a variety of sympathomimetic amines, as well as responses to the selective DA_1 agonist SKF 38393. Based upon these results, it was concluded that a sympathetic component, possibly mediated via the DA_1-type receptor, contributes to carrageenin-induced hyperalgesia [10]. A sympathetic hyperalgesic component has also been shown in other animal models [11, 12], although the receptors involved appear to depend upon the model or the animal species or both. Thus, the afferent fibres innervating rat neuroma were excited by sympathomimetic amines stimulating alpha-adrenoceptors [13].

Cytokines and the release of hyperalgesic mediators

Although the final hyperalgesic mediator might be a PG or a sympathomimetic amine, the release of these agents is usually preceded by the release of other mediators. The presence of foreign material in tissue or its injury causes an early response that can be considered as an alarm reaction in which resident macrophages appear to play a pivotal role in the development of acute inflammation [14]. At the onset of the inflammatory response the macrophage may act as an 'alarm cell', signalling the presence of foreign or deleterious stimuli via the release of cytokines. With the development of the inflammatory response, migrating cells such as polmorphonuclear leukocytes, macrophages, eosinophils and lymphocytes play an amplifying role. The actions of well-established inflammatory mediators, such as bradykinin and PGs, trigger local responses, reflected by the cardinal inflammatory symptoms and fever which assure the perception of an ongoing tissue injury and initiate defence mechanisms and reparative processes.

Over the past ten years or so it has become clear that in inflammatory responses, the release of hyperalgesic mediators is secondary to the release of proinflammatory cytokines. In this context, the release of cytokines appears to constitute a link between cellular injury and/or the recognition of 'non-self' and the liberation of the established mediators responsible for the development of local and systemic inflammatory signs and symptoms.

Interleukin-1 beta as a potent hyperalgesic agent

It had been known for some years that IL-1 was a potent inducer of PGs [15], which sensitise nociceptors [16]. The availability of human recombinant (h.r.) IL-1α and IL-1β [17] prompted the testing of these molecules for hyperalgesic (nociceptive) activity in a rat-paw pressure test [2]. Injection of IL-1β (at sub-picogram doses) into one paw (intraplantar, i.pl.) evoked a dose-dependent hyperalgesia in both paws (except for the smallest dose tested, which evoked ipsilateral hyperalgesia). This result was interpreted as indicating a systemic distribution of the tiny quantities of injected IL-1β since bilateral hyperalgesia also resulted from intraperitoneal (i.p.) injections of very small amounts of IL-1β [2]. An alternative explanation is that the injected IL-1β either stimulated release of another soluble mediator, or stimulated afferent nerves at the site of injection, or both. The hyperalgesic activity of IL-1β (injected i.pl.) was confirmed in the same model of mechanical hyperalgesia [4], but not in a different one [21], and was confirmed in models of thermal hyperalgesia [21, 22].

Although some three thousand times less potent than h.r. IL-1β, h.r. IL-1α still evoked hyperalgesia at sub-nanogram doses [2]. Since in most animal models, including those in rats, h.r. IL-1α and IL-1β have similar potencies for the IL-1 receptor (type I) that transduces IL-1 responses (see [1] and [2] for references), this difference may indicate that the IL-1 receptor that mediates hyperalgesia is a novel one with a higher affinity for IL-1β than for IL-1α. Alternatively, it might be a consequence of human IL-1α being a poorer ligand than human IL-1β for rat IL-1 receptors. Certain cytokines are known to exhibit species preference or specificity [18–20]. To date, rat cytokines, including rat IL-1α, have not been tested for hyperalgesic activity in rats.

Role of cyclo-oxygenase products in IL-1 induced hyperalgesia

Local pre-treatment with a large dose of indomethacin (a non-steroidal anti-inflammatory drug that inhibits cyclo-oxygenase [23]) markedly attenuated the develop-

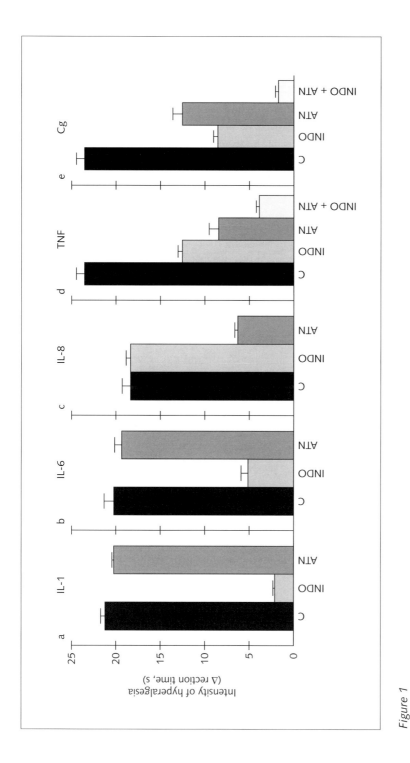

Figure 1

Effect of indomethacin and atenolol on responses to hyperalgesic agents.
Inhibition of hyperalgesic responses measured 3 h after injection (100 μl, i.pl.) of (a) IL-1β (IL-1, 0.5 pg), (b) IL-6 (1 ng), (c) IL-8 (100 pg), TNFα (TNF, 2.5 pg) and (e) carrageenin (Cg, 100 μg) by drugs given (100 μl, i.pl.) 30 min before the hyperalgesic agents: C = saline, INDO = indomethacin (100 μg), K(D)PT = Lys-D-Pro-Thr (200 μg), ATN = atenolol (25 μg). Means ± s.e.m. in groups of 5 rats are shown.

ment of IL-1β-evoked hyperalgesia in the rat model of mechanical hyperalgesia described above (Fig. 1: first panel), although a smaller dose of indomethacin (given orally) was without effect [4]. In a different model, the acetylcholine-induced pain reflex in the rabbit perfused isolated ear, the (similar) hyperalgesic effects of both h.r. IL-1α and IL-1β were abolished by the cyclo-oxygenase inhibitor diclofenac-Na [3]. The consensus of the above data is that local release by IL-1 of cyclo-oxygenase products, such as PGs, in the vicinity of nociceptors contributes to IL-1-evoked hyperalgesia.

Other proinflammatory cytokines as hyperalgesic agents

In addition to IL-1, the cytokines TNFα, IL-6 and IL-8 are generally regarded as proinflammatory, although IL-6 has anti-inflammatory as well as proinflammatory actions [24, 25]. Given the remarkably potent hyperalgesic activity of IL-1, it was not long before these other cytokines were tested in the rat paw pressure test that had first identified IL-1 as a hyperalgesic agent. When injected i.pl., h.r. TNFα, IL-6 and IL-8 were also shown to possess hyperalgesic activities, evoking bilateral hyperalgesia, although there were qualitative and quantitative differences in the hyperalgesic responses to the cytokines [26, 27]. These cytokines, like IL-1β, evoked hyperalgesia at doses which did not cause oedema.

Qualitatively, hyperalgesic responses to IL-8 were similar to responses to IL-1β. The responses were of fast onset with the intensity of hyperalgesia reaching a plateau within 60 min of injection and starting to decline within six hours [2, 26]. Responses to TNFα and IL-6 were of slower onset with the intensity of hyperalgesia reaching a plateau within two to three hours of injection; responses to IL-6 were maintained at six hours whereas responses to TNFα had begun to decline at six hours after injection [27]. The responses to all the cytokines returned to pre-injection values within 24 h.

Quantitatively, the doses of the four cytokines that evoked maximum hyperalgesic effects were: IL-1β (0.5 pg), TNFα (2.5 pg), IL-8 (100 pg), IL-6 (1000 pg), giving an order of potency of IL-1β > TNFα >> IL-8 >> IL-6 for these human cytokines in rats. Whether this order of potency reflects the order of potency of the endogenous cytokines of the rat is unknown. As noted above, certain cytokines exhibit species preference or specificity [18–20] and the native cytokines remain to be tested.

Mechanisms underlying the hyperalgesic activities of IL-1β, IL-6, IL-8 and TNFα
The relative contributions of cyclo-oxygenase products and the sympathetic nervous system to the hyperalgesic activities of IL-1β, IL-6, IL-8 and TNFα (given i.pl.) were

investigated in experiments in which the hyperalgesic responses to the four cytokines were measured subsequent to the administration of indomethacin, the β-adrenoceptor antagonist atenolol, or both (Fig. 1). The effects of indomethacin and atenolol on hyperalgesic responses to the inflammatory agent carrageenin were also tested. As can be seen from Figure 1, indomethacin abolished the response to IL-1β, markedly attenuated the response to IL-6, reduced by about 50% responses to TNFα and carrageenin, but did not affect the response to IL-8. In contrast, atenolol did not affect responses to IL-1β and IL-6, markedly attenuated the responses to IL-8 and TNFα, and reduced by about 50% the response to carrageenin. The combination of indomethacin and atenolol abolished responses to TNFα and carrageenin (Fig. 1).

The above data, together with other data [2, 27], suggest that IL-1β and IL-6 caused hyperalgesia by releasing cyclo-oxygenase products. In the case of IL-1β, by inducing gene-expression of cyclo-oxgenase-2 (COX-2) [28] and phospholipase A_2 [29], and in the case of IL-6 by inducing arachidonic acid release [24, 25]. In contrast to IL-1β, IL-8 caused hyperalgesia by releasing sympathomimetic amines. The capacity of both indomethacin and atenolol to inhibit responses to TNFα and carrageenin suggests a role for both cyclo-oxygenase products and sympathomimetic amines in the mediation of their hyperalgesic effects.

A cascade of release of hyperalgesic cytokines

A property of several cytokines is their capacity to induce their own production, that of other cytokines, or both; also, certain cytokines can inhibit the production of other cytokines or down-regulate their receptor numbers [24]. This complex web of interactions is sometimes referred to as the cytokine network. For example, TNFα induces production of IL-1 [30] and IL-1 induces the production of IL-1 [31], IL-6 [32], and IL-8 [33]. In addition, IL-6 suppresses IL-1 production, *in vitro*, by monocytes/macrophages stimulated with bacterial endotoxin (lipopolysaccharide, LPS) or TNFα [34]. IL-6 induces production, *in vivo*, of anti-inflammatory proteins: IL-1 receptor antagonist and soluble tumour necrosis factor receptor [35].

A considerable body of evidence indicates that the sequence of events in the production of proinflammatory cytokines, following parenteral administration of an inflammatory stimuli such as bacteria, LPS, or turpentine is that TNFα production is induced, and that this cytokine induces production of IL-1. This then induces production of IL-6 [32, 36] and IL-8 [33], although in some models of inflammation the production of IL-6 appears to be under the control of TNFα [37] rather than IL-1 [38]. To investigate the sequence of cytokine release that occurs during hyperalgesic responses to the inflammatory agent carrageenin in rat paws, the effects of neutralising anti-cytokine sera on hyperalgesic responses were investigated [27].

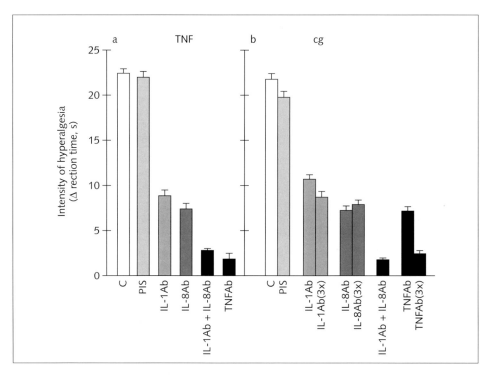

Figure 2
Effect of anti-cytokine sera on hyperalgesic responses to TNFα and carrageenin.
Effect of anti-cytokine sera on the hyperalgesic responses measured 3 h after injection (100 µl, i.pl.) of (a) TNFα (2.5 pg) and (b) carrageenin (100 µg). Panel (a) sheep anti-rat cytokine sera were incubated for 15 min with the TNFα before injection of the mixture (final volume = 100 µl). Panel (b) sheep anti-rat cytokine sera (50 µl, except where x3 = 150 µl is indicated, in a final volume of 150 µl) were injected 30 min before carrageenin. C = saline, PIS = pre-immune normal sheep serum, IL-1Ab = sheep anti-IL-1β serum, IL-8Ab = sheep anti-IL-8 serum, TNFAb = sheep anti-TNFα serum. Means ± s.e.m. in groups of 5 rats are shown.

The pivotal role of TNFα

From panel (a) of Figure 2 it can be seen that hyperalgesic responses to TNFα were inhibited (by ≥ 50%) by antisera neutralising IL-1β or IL-8 and effectively abolished by the combination of anti-IL-1β and anti-IL-8 sera. From panel (b) of the same figure it can be seen that hyperalgesic responses to carrageenin were similarly attenuated by antisera neutralising IL-1β or IL-8 and effectively abolished by either an anti-TNFα serum or the combination of anti-IL-1β and anti-IL-8 sera. These data, taken together with the data shown in Figure 1 (and described above) and other data [26, 27], are consistent with the existence of a cascade of cytokine production in which the inflammatory stimulus carrageenin induces production of TNFα, which activates two pathways. One pathway involves production of IL-1β and IL-6, which release cyclo-oxygenase products, and the other involves production of IL-8, which releases sympathomimetic amines [26, 27]. Thus, in this model of inflammatory hyperalgesia, the production of IL-6 and IL-8 appears to be under the control of TNFα, rather than IL-1β.

Data from a severe model of (chronic) inflammatory hyperalgesia, resulting from the injection (i.pl.) of Freund's complete adjuvant, also provided evidence for a role of TNFα-induced IL-1β production in the early phase of the inflammatory hyperalgesia [39]. The possible role of IL-6 and IL-8, and the sequence of their release, relative to that of TNFα and IL-1β, in this model of inflammatory hyperalgesia has not yet been tested.

The sequence of release of IL-1β and IL-6

The sequence of production of IL-1β and IL-6 was investigated in experiments in which the hyperalgesic responses to these cytokines were measured subsequent to the administration of antisera neutralising either IL-1β or IL-6, or the specific IL-1 receptor antagonist, IL-1ra (Fig. 3). The hyperalgesic effect of IL-1β was inhibited by pre-treatment with an anti-IL-β serum and by IL-1ra (as expected) and the hyperalgesic effect of IL-6 was inhibited by pre-treatment with an anti-IL-6 serum (as expected). However, an unexpected finding was the inhibition of IL-6-induced hyperalgesia by the anti-IL-β serum and by IL-1ra (Fig. 3). These data are consistent with IL-1β-induced production of IL-6. Although the converse, i.e. IL-1-induced production of IL-6, occurs *in vitro* [32] and *in vivo* [36], IL-6 was not found to induce production of IL-1β *in vitro* by human peripheral blood mononuclear cells (S. Poole, unpublished data). The effect of rat sequence IL-6 on IL-1β production by rat macrophages has not been tested. The data described above is consistent with the following sequence of release of cytokines and other hyperalgesic mediators:

stimulus (e.g. carrageenin) → TNFα → IL-6 → IL-1β (cyclo-oxygenase products
                                    ↓
                                  IL-8
                                    ↓
                        sympathomimetic amines

The placing of IL-6, which has more anti-inflammatory actions than proinflammatory ones [24, 25], between the proinflammatory mediators TNFα and IL-1β might appear incongruous but it is possible that, *in vivo*, in the presence of the full reper-

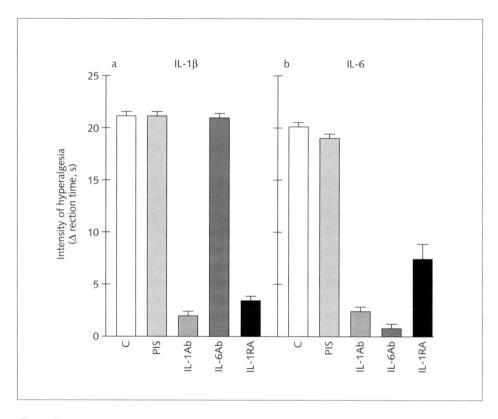

Figure 3
Effect of anti-cytokine sera and IL-1ra on hyperalgesic responses to IL-1β and IL-6.
Effect of anti-cytokine sera and the IL-1 receptor antagonist, IL-1ra, on the hyperalgesic
responses measured 3 h after injection (100 µl, i.pl.) of (a) IL-1β (0.5 pg) and (b) IL-6 (1 ng).
Sheep anti-rat cytokine sera (100 µl) or IL-1ra (20 pg in 100 µl) were injected 30 min before
the cytokines. C = saline, PIS = pre-immune normal sheep serum, IL-1Ab = sheep anti-IL-1β
serum, IL-8Ab = sheep anti-IL-8 serum, TNFAb = sheep anti-TNFα serum. Means ± s.e.m. in
groups of 5 rats are shown.

toire of cells and mediators involved in inflammatory hyperalgesia, IL-6 has the
capacity to induce IL-1 production. This scenario has been postulated to be the case
in cytokine-mediated pyrogenic responses in rats in which proinflammatory stimuli
induce production of IL-6 in the periphery (secondary to the production of TNFα
and IL-1β) and that IL-6 induces production of IL-1 in the brain [36, 40]. Clearly,
further experiments, in which native sequence cytokines (and antibodies to them)
are injected in rats, are required to elucidate the precise sequence of events in the
hyperalgesic pathway that involves IL-1β, IL-6 and PGs.

Bradykinin initiates cytokine-mediated inflammatory hyperalgesia

Bradykinin produces overt pain in man when instilled into the cantharidin blister base [41], when injected into the abdominal cavity [42], or into the cephalic, brachial vein previously sensitised with serotonin [43]. These effects result from activation of nociceptors but bradykinin also sensitises nociceptors, which leads to the development of inflammatory hyperalgesia. The immediate (direct) effect of bradykinin has been studied extensively in both behavioural and electro-physiological models (see [44] for references) and appears to result from the activation of high threshold nociceptors associated with C fibres. The delayed and long-lasting hyperalgesic effect of bradykinin, in contrast, has received rather less attention, although there is good evidence for a role for bradykinin in a number of different models of inflammatory hyperalgesia [45–48] and a specific bradykinin B_2 receptor antagonist, HOE 140, has been shown to inhibit the delayed hyperalgesic effect of bradykinin. HOE 140 was anti-hyperalgesic in experimental models of inflammatory pain, especially in carrageenin-induced hyperalgesia [49]. Given the capacity of the bradykinin B_2 antagonist HOE 140 to inhibit carrageenin-evoked inflammatory hyperalgesia and a report that bradykinin evoked the release of TNFα and IL-1 from macrophage monolayers [50], it was a logical step to investigate the possibility that bradykinin was involved in the cytokine-mediated hyperalgesic pathways activated by carrageenin described above [26, 27].

Hyperalgesic responses to bradykinin were inhibited by antisera neutralising IL-1β, IL-6 or IL-8 and abolished by an antiserum neutralising TNFα (Fig. 4). The neutralising effects of antisera neutralising IL-1β and IL-6 were not additive, but the combinations of anti-IL-1β plus anti-IL-8 sera and of anti-IL-6 plus anti-IL-8 sera were additive and both combinations abolished hyperalgesic responses to bradykinin (Fig. 4). In contrast to the abolition of bradykinin-evoked hyperalgesia by pretreatment with anti-TNFα serum, TNFα-evoked hyperalgesia was not inhibited by the bradykinin B_2 receptor antagonist, HOE 140, suggesting that bradykinin induced production of TNFα and not vice-versa [41]. Considered together with the report that bradykinin induced production of TNF and IL-1 in cultures of murine macrophage cell lines [50] these data suggest that bradykinin initiates the cascade of cytokines by stimulating the production of TNFα. The TNFα then induces production of: (i) IL-6 and IL-1β, which stimulate the production of cyclo-oxygenase products, and (ii) IL-8, which stimulates the production of sympathomimetics [26, 27, 44].

A study contemporary with the one described above showed that the (bilateral) thermal hyperalgesia evoked by IL-1β (injected i.pl.), but not the (unilateral) hyperalgesia evoked by TNFα (injected i.pl.), was mediated by bradykinin B_1 receptors [22]. This finding and data from other models [22, 51] suggests roles for both types of bradykinin receptor in a complex network of hyperalgesic mediators in which bradykinin can induce cytokines and vice-versa. It has been suggested that B_2 recep-

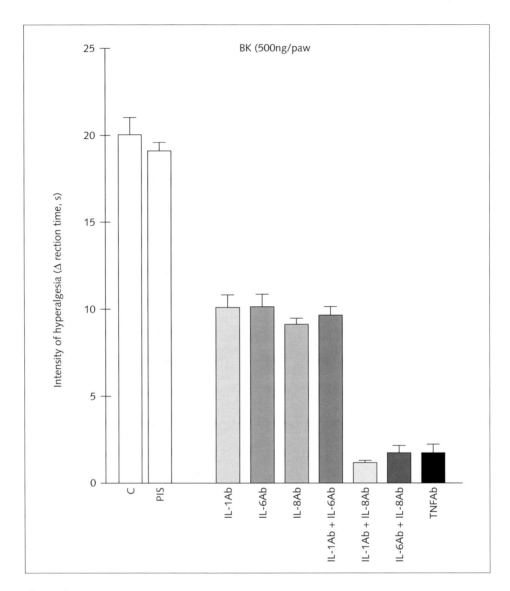

Figure 4

Figure 4 Effect of anti-cytokine sera on hyperalgesic responses to bradykinin.

Effect of anti-cytokine sera on the hyperalgesic responses measured 3 h after injection (in 100 (l, i.pl.) of bradykinin (500 ng). Sheep anti-rat cytokine sera (50 (l in a final volume of 100 (l) were injected 30 min before carrageenin. C = saline, PIS = pre-immune normal sheep serum, IL-1Ab = sheep anti-IL-1β serum, IL-6Ab = sheep anti-IL-6 serum, IL-8Ab = sheep anti-IL-8 serum, TNFAb = sheep anti-TNFβ serum. Means ± s.e.m. in groups of 5 rats are shown.

tors may play a more significant part in the earlier stages of inflammatory pain, with B1 receptors maintaining the hyperalgesic state during inflammation and injury [52]. B_2 receptors have been localised to sensory neurones [53, 54] whereas B_1 receptors are located on cells other than sensory neurones [55]. Knowledge of the precise location of the two receptor types (e.g. on nociceptive neurones, macrophages, vascular smooth muscle and synovial cells) and of the conditions required for their expression should improve our understanding of the kinin/cytokine pathways.

When bradykinin is incorporated into the cascade of hyperalgesic mediators proposed above, the sequence becomes:

$$\text{stimulus (e.g. carrageenin)} \rightarrow \text{bradykinin} \rightarrow \text{TNF}\alpha \rightarrow \text{IL-6} \rightarrow \text{IL-1}\beta \rightarrow \text{cyclo-oxygenase}$$

$$(B_2) (B_1 ?) \quad \downarrow \qquad\qquad \downarrow \qquad\qquad \text{products}$$

$$\text{IL-8} \qquad\qquad \text{bradykinin}$$

$$\downarrow \qquad\qquad (B_1)$$

$$\text{sympathomimetic}$$

$$\text{amines}$$

Although bradykinin initiates the cascade of cytokines by stimulating the production of TNFα in response to stimuli such as carrageenin or a small dose of LPS (1 μg) [44], the cytokine cascade can be activated independently of bradykinin if the hyperalgesic stimulus is of sufficient magnitude. Thus, a larger dose of LPS (5 μg) evoked hyperalgesia that was not inhibited by the bradykinin B_2 antagonist HOE 140 [44].

There is substantial literature showing that carrageenin and LPS activate the plasma kinin system [56, 57] and that LPS is a potent, 'direct' activator of cytokine production, especially from cells of the monocyte/macrophage lineage. Therefore, the contribution of bradykinin to the development of inflammatory hyperalgesia in some pathological processes may well be overshadowed by either 'direct' stimulation of cytokine production by stimuli such as LPS or by other intermediates in hyperalgesic pathways. Consequently, the usefulness of bradykinin antagonists as anti-hyperalgesics will depend upon the relative contribution of bradykinin to the release of cytokines and other hyperalgesic mediators, with bradykinin antagonists most likely to be useful in conditions such as mumps, pancreatitis, intense burns, and Gram-negative infections in which kinin systems are activated.

Anti-inflammatory cytokines limit cytokine-mediated inflammatory hyperalgesia

In recent years a number of 'anti-inflammatory' cytokines have been described which inhibit the production of cytokines that are generally regarded as proinflammatory. For example, the T cell-derived cytokine IL-4 has coordinated anti-inflammatory effects by suppressing IL-1 production and up-regulating production of the IL-1 receptor antagonist IL-1ra by LPS-stimulated human monocytes [58, 59]. Consistent with these findings is an earlier study in which IL-4 down-regulated the expression of CD14 (a putative LPS receptor [60]) in human monocytes [61]. Such results emphasise the integrated nature of cytokine production and interaction.

Another 'antagonist cytokine' is IL-10, a product of (murine) Th2 lymphocytes and monocytes. IL-10 inhibits production of cytokines by murine Th1 lymphocytes [62] and is thought to play a role in inhibiting delayed type hypersensitivity responses [63, 64] and in suppressing macrophage functions, such as class II expression [65], adhesion [66], and the synthesis of cytokines (including IL-1, IL-6, IL-8, granulocyte colony stimulating factor (G-CSF), granulocyte-macrophage colony stimulating factor (GM-CSF) and TNFα) [66–68]. Also, IL-10 up-regulates the expression of IL-1ra [69].

The capacities of IL-4, a neutralising monoclonal antibody to IL-4, IL-10, a neutralising monoclonal antibody to IL-10, and IL-1ra to modulate (cytokine-mediated) hyperalgesic responses to carrageenin are shown in Figure 5. The effects of one of these anti-inflammatory cytokines, IL-10, to also diminish hyperalgesic responses to bradykinin and proinflammatory cytokines has been described previously [71]. IL-4, IL-10 and IL-1ra all markedly attenuated hyperalgesic responses to carrageenin (100 µg: the smallest dose that evoked a maximum response, Fig. 5, panel (a)). In contrast, neutralising monoclonal antibodies to IL-4 and IL-10 potentiated hyperalgesic responses to a sub-maximum dose of carrageenin (10 µg). These data provide strong evidence that IL-4, IL-10 and IL-1ra limit (cytokine-mediated) hyperalgesic responses to carrageenin. In the case of IL-10, inflammatory hyperalgesia was limited by two mechanisms: inhibition of cytokine production and inhibition of IL-1β-evoked PGE_2 production, with the latter effect mediated not via IL-10-induced IL-1ra [71] but by suppression by IL-10 of the inducible form of cyclo-oxygenase, COX-2 (PG H Synthase-2) [71, 72].

Role of lipocortin-1 in the anti-hyperalgesic actions of glucocorticoids

It is now well established that glucocorticoid drugs, e.g. dexamethasone, inhibit both the early and late changes that contribute to the inflammatory process. A glucocorticoid-inducible protein of 37 kDa, lipocortin-1 (LC-1), has been identified as an endogenous mediator of the anti-inflammatory actions of glucocorticoids [73]. Although human LC-1 comprises 346 amino acids, the N-terminal polypeptide, LC-1$_{1-188}$, mimics a variety of the anti-inflammatory effects of glucocorticoids [74] and an N-terminal peptide comprising of just 25 amino acids, LC-1$_{2-26}$, has also been shown to mimic the anti-inflammatory effects of LC-1 [75]. LC-1$_{2-26}$ was

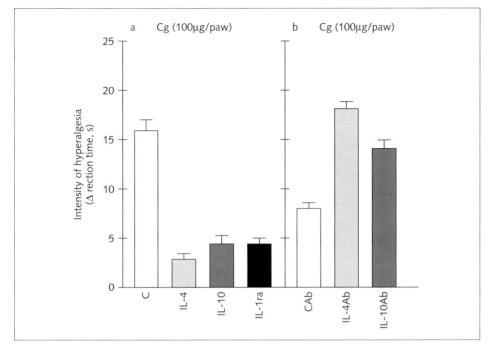

Figure 5
Anti-inflammatory cytokines inhibit hyperalgesic responses to carrageenin.
Panel (a) effect of murine IL-4 (10 ng), IL-10 (10 ng) and IL-1ra (20 pg), on hyperalgesic responses measured 3 h after injection (100 μl, i.pl.) of carrageenin (100 μg). Panel (b) effect of monoclonal antibodies (MAbs) to ovalbumin, murine IL-4 and murine IL-10 on hyperalgesic responses measured 3 h after injection (100 μl, i.pl.) of carrageenin (10 μg). Cytokines and MAbs were injected 30 min before carrageenin. C = saline, CAb = control MAb to ovalbumin (150 μg in 150 μl), IL-4Ab = MAb to IL-4 BVDG (50 μg 150 μl i.pl.), IL-10Ab = MAb to IL-10 SXC-1 (150 μg in 50 μl i.pl.). Means ± s.e.m. in groups of 5 rats are shown.

about 200 times less active than LC-1 on a molar basis although both molecules gave maximum inhibition of IL-1-induced leukocyte migration [75] and, in mice, immunoneutralisation of endogenous LC-1 with an antiserum to LC-1$_{2-26}$, designated LCPS1, exacerbated the acute inflammatory response to zymosan [76].

Recently, the effects of LC-1$_{2-26}$, LCPS1 and the glucocorticoid dexamethasone on the cascade of endogenous mediators that contribute to carrageenin-evoked inflammatory hyperalgesia in rat paws were investigated [77]. Hyperalgesic responses to carrageenin, bradykinin, TNFα, and IL-1β, but not responses to PGE$_2$, were inhibited by prior treatment with dexamethasone or LC-1$_{2-26}$ (Fig. 6, panel (a)). Further, the inhibition of hyperalgesic responses to bradykinin and IL-1β by

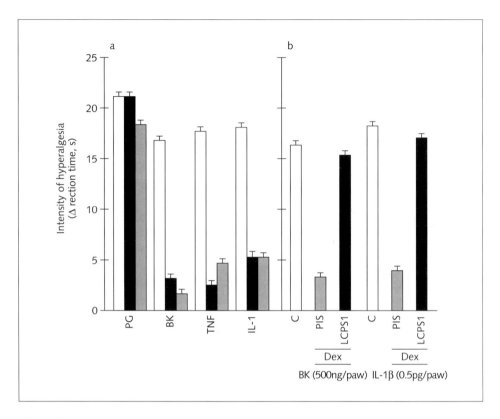

Figure 6
Lipocortin mediates the anti-hyperalgesic effect of dexamethasone.
Panel (a) effect of dexamethasone and LC-1$_{2-26}$ on hyperalgesic responses measured 3 h after injection (100 µl, i.pl.) of PGE$_2$ (PG, 100 ng), bradykinin (500 ng), TNFα (TNF, 2.5 pg) and IL-1β (IL-1, 0.5 pg). Dexamethasone (DEX, 0.5 mg kg^{-1}, 0.2 ml, injected subcutaneously, s.c.) and LC-1$_{2-26}$ (LC, 100 µg in 100 µl, i.pl.) were given 1 h before hyperalgesic substances. Panel (b) abolition by LCPS1 of the anti-hyperalgesic effect of dexamethasone. Responses were measured 3 h after injection (in 100 µl, i.pl.) of bradykinin (BK, 500 ng) and IL-1β (IL-1, 0.5 pg). Dexamethasone (DEX, 0.5 mg kg^{-1}, s.c.) or PBS (0.5 ml kg^{-1}, s.c.) was given 1 h before hyperalgesic substances. LCPS1 (0.5 ml kg^{-1}, filled columns), pre-immune serum (PIS, 0.5 ml kg^{-1}, stippled columns) or no pre-treatment (C, open columns) was given, s.c., 24 h and 1 h before dexamethasone. Means ± s.e.m. in groups of 5 rats are shown.

dexamethasone was reversed by LCPS1 (Fig. 6, panel (b)). In other experiments, dexamethasone inhibited hyperalgesic responses to carrageenin, arachidonic acid plus IL-1β and IL-6 but not hyperalgesic responses to IL-8 and dopamine [77]. Taken together with the results described above (and shown in Fig. 6), these findings are consistent with the existence of the two hyperalgesic pathways postulated above, with dexamethasone inhibiting the production of PGs and other eicosanoids [78, 79], TNFα [80], IL-1β [81], and IL-6 [82] to block one pathway, and inhibiting the production of TNFα [80] and IL-8 [83] to block the other pathway.

The capacity of LCPS1 to reverse the inhibition by dexamethasone of the hyperalgesic responses to bradykinin and IL-1β, and the finding that hyperalgesic responses to bradykinin, TNFα and IL-1β and arachidonic acid plus IL-1β were inhibited by prior treatment with LC-1$_{2-26}$, suggest that endogenous LC-1 mediated the anti-hyperalgesic effect of dexamethasone and that this biological activity of LC-1 resides within the peptide LC-1$_{2-26}$. These suggestions are in agreement with the data from the other models described above [75, 76].

Dexamethasone abolished, whereas LC-1$_{2-26}$ only partially inhibited, the production of TNFα by J774 murine macrophage cells stimulated with LPS, suggesting that the inhibitory activity of dexamethasone on TNFα production was only partially mediated by LC-1 [44]. This suggestion is supported by the finding that an antiserum to LC-1$_{2-26}$ only partially reversed the inhibitory effect of dexamethasone on TNFα release by J774 cells stimulated with LPS [77]. Dexamethasone and other glucocorticoids are now known to have an important biological activity in addition to those described above. This is the capacity to stimulate production of IκBα, which binds to and inhibits NF-κB, a transcription factor that plays a central role in the induction of a number of cytokine genes, including TNFα, IL-1, IL-2, IL-3, IL-6, IL-8, interferon-γ (IFNγ) and G-CSF [84, 85]. Several of these genes are also regulated by another transcription factor, AP-1 [86–88], which synergises with NF-κB [89]. The inhibition by glucocorticoids of the activities of both NF-κB and AP-1 provides additional mechanisms to explain the potent immunosuppressive, anti-inflammatory and anti-hyperalgesic effects of these drugs.

The finding that LC-1$_{2-26}$ abolished the inflammatory hyperalgesia mediated by cytokines and an antiserum to this peptide abolished the analgesic effect of dexamethasone *in vivo* suggests that the anti-hyperalgesic effect of glucocorticoids in this model is entirely dependent upon LC-1 release [77]. LC-1$_{2-26}$ may also have affected events other than the release of proinflammatory cytokines, such as inhibition of the induction of (the inducible) cyclo-oxygenase enzyme (COX-2) responsible for the PG production that contributes to inflammatory hyperalgesia. Consistent with this possibility was the finding that arachidonic acid by itself was not hyperalgesic but potentiated the hyperalgesic effect of IL-1β, which is known to induce COX-2 [28]. Further, both dexamethasone and LC-1$_{2-26}$ strongly inhibited this potentiation, and LC-1 abolished the production of PGE$_2$ by J774 cells stimulated with LPS. Although inhibition of phospholipase A$_2$ by dexamethasone and LC-1$_{2-26}$ is believed to underlie the anti-inflammatory effects of dexamethasone and LC-1 [78, 79], the above data suggest that in inflammatory hyperalgesia inhibition of the induction of COX-2 (rather than phospholipase A$_2$) by dexamethasone and LC-1$_{2-26}$ accounts for the anti-hyperalgesic effects of these agents. In addition, LC-1/LC-1$_{2-26}$ may have a role in the effects of glucocorticoids on NF-κB and AP-1. Taken together, the above data indicate that the analgesic effect of glucocorticoids in cytokine-mediated inflammatory hyperalgesia, in the absence of oedema formation and leukocyte migration, results from the induction of LC-1. This is responsible for the inhibition of the production of hyperalgesic cytokines and inhibition of the production of eicosanoids by COX-2.

Novel tripeptide antagonists of hyperalgesic responses involving IL-1β

The IL-1β analogue: Lys-D-Pro-Thr

The first report that IL-1β was a potent hyperalgesic agent also described a tripeptide analogue of IL-1β that inhibited hyperalgesic responses to IL-1β but not those to IL-1α [2]. The tripeptide, Lys-D-Pro-Thr, derived from IL-1β$^{193-195}$ (Lys^{193}-Pro-Thr^{195}) [2], did not antagonise responses to IL-1β in an (*in vitro*) EL-4 thymoma conversion assay (for IL-1) or in the (*in vivo*) rabbit pyrogen test [2]. The possibility that the anti-hyperalgesic effect of Lys-D-Pro-Thr was mediated centrally was excluded because the peptide did not antagonise PGE$_2$-induced hyperalgesia and was not effective in a 'hot-plate test', unlike centrally acting analgesic drugs such as morphine [2].

The dose of Lys-D-Pro-Thr (1.3 mg kg^{-1} = 3.8 μmol kg^{-1}) that inhibited hyperalgesia in response to IL-1β also inhibited the response to carrageenin, but not the response to PGE$_2$ (Fig. 7). The maximum anti-hyperalgesic effect of Lys-D-Pro-Thr was similar to that of indomethacin [5, 26, 27, 91]. The residual hyperalgesia evoked by carrageenin was likely to have been due to the sympathetic component present in carrageenin-evoked hyperalgesia [10] since the combination of the adrenergic neurone blocking agent guanethidine with Lys-D-Pro-Thr abolished carrageenin-evoked hyperalgesia [2]. Subsequently it was shown (as noted above) that the sympathetic component of carrageenin-evoked hyperalgesia was activated by IL-8 [26], the production of which was induced by TNFα [27]. In addition to hyperalgesic responses to IL-1β and carrageenin, Lys-D-Pro-Thr also inhibited hyperalgesic responses to IL-6 and TNFα, which involve IL-1β-induced release of PGs [2, 27, 44]. Although the effect of Lys-D-Pro-Thr was not additive with that of indomethacin [27], Lys-D-Pro-Thr is not an inhibitor of cyclo-oxygenase [2].

Inhibition by Lys-D-Pro-Thr of IL-1β-evoked mechanical hyperalgesia was soon confirmed by others [4] and Lys-D-Pro-Thr has now been shown to be a highly effective inhibitor of (usually PG-dependent) responses involving IL-1β. For example, Lys-D-Pro-Thr reversed the inhibition by IL-1β of (electrically-stimulated) long term potentiation in the mossy fibre-CA3 pathway of mouse hippocampal slice preparations [92] and inhibited IL-1β-induced augmentation of capsaicin-induced release of

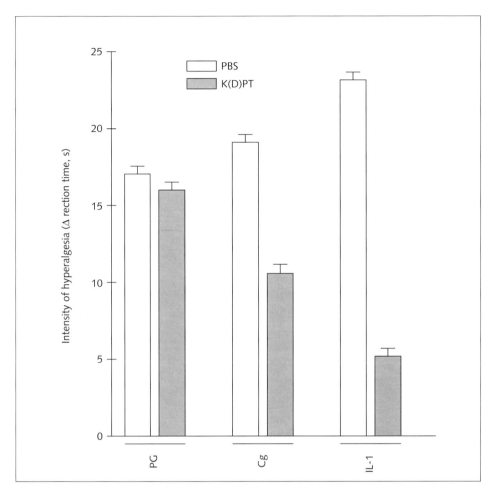

Figure 7
Inhibition by Lys-D-Pro-Thr of IL-1β-mediated hyperalgesic responses.
Effect of Lys-D-Pro-Thr (K(D)PT, 1.3 mg kg^{-1} = 3.8 (mol kg^{-1}, in 0.3 ml, injected intraperi-
toneally, i.p., 30 min before the hyperalgesic agents) on hyperalgesic responses measured 3
h after injection (100 µl, i.pl.) of PGE$_2$ (PG, 100 ng), carrageenin (Cg, 100 µg), and IL-1β (0.5
pg). Means ± s.e.m. in groups of 5 rats are shown. PBS = phosphate buffered saline.

calcitonin gene related peptide from capsaicin-sensitive nerves in the trachea (a PG-dependent response) [93]. Also, Lys-D-Pro-Thr (in common with IL-1ra) inhibited [des-Arg^9]BK-induced (PG-dependent) mechanical hyperalgesia in rat knee joints [94]. The specificity of Lys-D-Pro-Thr as an inhibitor of (PG-dependent) IL-1β responses only involving nervous tissue is suggested by the lack of effect of Lys-D-Pro-Thr on the (PG-dependent) IL-1β-evoked relaxation of rabbit isolated mesenteric artery [95].

α-MSH and its analogues

α-MSH and its metabolically stable analogue [Nl⁴,D-Phe⁷]α-MSH inhibit a number of responses to IL-1β (see [1] and [96] for references) including mechanical hyperalgesia [4]. Also, the C-terminal peptide of α-MSH, α-MSH[11-13] (Lys[11]-Pro-Val[13]), is anti-pyretic against leukocyte pyrogen [97], of which IL-1β is a major component [98], and is reported to have antiinflammatory activity [99, 100].

The structural similarity between the C-terminus of α-MSH[11-13] (Lys[11]-Pro-Val[13]) and the IL-1β analogue Lys-D-Pro-Thr prompted a study of the structure versus anti-hyperalgesic activity against IL-1β and PGE$_2$ of a series of peptides related to α-MSH and Lys-D-Pro-Thr [96]. Hyperalgesic responses to IL-1β were inhibited in a dose-dependent manner by peptides with the following order of potency: [Nl⁴,D-Phe⁷]α-MSH > α-MSH > Lys-D-Pro-Val > Lys-Pro-Val > Lys-D-Pro-Thr > D-Lys-Pro-Thr. The marked loss in anti-hyperalgesic activity that resulted from deletion of the C-terminal peptide Lys[11]-Pro-Val[13] from α-MSH and [Nl⁴,D-Phe⁷]α-MSH, taken together with the anti-hyperalgesic activity of Lys-Pro-Val, point to its importance in the activities of the full-length peptides. The above results are consistent with an earlier study of the anti-pyretic effect (presumably against IL-1β) of α-MSH analogues with truncated N-termini [101]. The residual activity of [Nl⁴,D-Phe⁷]α-MSH[1-10] and α-MSH[1–10] suggests an additional site with anti-hyperalgesic activity (against IL-1β and PGE$_2$) within these decapeptides.

Hyperalgesic responses to PGE$_2$ were inhibited in a dose-dependent manner by the following peptides, with the same order of potency as against IL-1β: [Nl⁴,D-Phe⁷]α-MSH > α-MSH > Lys-D-Pro-Val > Lys-Pro-Val. Lys-D-Pro-Thr and D-Lys-Pro-Thr were not active against PGE$_2$, suggesting that the anti-hyperalgesic effect of the threonine compounds might be specific to IL-1β. A recent report that Lys-D-Pro-Val but not Lys-D-Pro-Thr inhibited hyperalgesic responses to thymulin [102] is consistent with the specificity for IL-1β of the threonine compounds.

The selective κ-opioid receptor antagonist, Nor-binaltorphimine (Nor-BNI), largely reversed the anti-hyperalgesic effects of [Nl⁴,D-Phe⁷]α-MSH, α-MSH, Lys-D-Pro-Val, and Lys-Pro-Val against both IL-1β and PGE$_2$, providing good evidence that the anti-hyperalgesic activities of these four peptides were mediated by endogenous opioids acting on κ-opioid receptors. This notion is consistent with a study in rats in which α-MSH and related peptides, given centrally, reduced responsiveness to pain, with α-MSH eliciting a behavioural profile similar to that produced by β-endorphin [103]. Also, in mice, the opioid receptor antagonist naloxone (given s.c.) prevented the analgesic action of α-MSH (given intracerebroventricularly) [104]. The lack of effect of Nor-BNI on the anti-hyperalgesic effects of Lys-D-Pro-Thr and

D-Lys-Pro-Thr indicates that these peptides were not working via κ-opioid receptors, a finding consistent with the lack of effect of naloxone on inhibition by Lys-D-Pro-Thr of IL-1β-evoked hyperalgesia [4]. Also consistent with the non-opioid mechanism of action of Lys-D-Pro-Thr is its failure to inhibit PGE$_2$-evoked hyperalgesia [2, 96], in contrast to morphine [91] and the finding that the antinociceptive activity of Lys-D-Pro-Val, but not that of Lys-D-Pro-Thr, was reversed by the opioid receptor antagonist, naloxone [105].

Despite the analgesic activity described for α-MSH injected centrally [103, 104], α-MSH, given i.v. showed no effect on PGE$_2$-evoked hyperalgesia in a hot-plate test, in contrast to morphine [4]. Likewise, Lys-D-Pro-Thr, Lys-Pro-Val and Lys-D-Pro-Val were not anti-hyperalgesic in a hot-plate test, in contrast to morphine ([2], S.H. Ferreira, unpublished data). These data indicate a peripheral rather than a central site of action for the peptides described above. The receptors mediating the anti-hyperalgesic effects of the peptides remain to be elucidated but appear distinct from receptors for IL-1 and α-MSH since Lys-D-Pro-Thr did not inhibit responses to IL-1β other than hyperalgesic responses [2, 96] and Lys-Pro-Val did not inhibit receptor binding of a radio-labelled analogue of α-MSH [106].

Conclusions

The field of 'cytokines in inflammatory hyperalgesia' is now ten years old and much has been learned (see Fig. 8). IL-1β has been shown to be a potent hyperalgesic agent which can be antagonised by small, orally active [105] peptides with therapeutic potential. Two hyperalgesic pathways have been identified which involve proinflammatory cytokines and other hyperalgesic mediators: inflammatory stimuli, such as carrageenin and LPS, induce the production of bradykinin, which stimulates the release of TNFα. The TNFα induces production of (i) IL-6 and IL-1β, which stimulate the production of cyclo-oxygenase products, and (ii) IL-8, which stimulates production of sympathomimetics. The capacity of IL-8, which is released by activated macrophages and endothelial cells, to cause hyperalgesia by a PG-independent mechanism that involves the sympathetic nervous system suggests that IL-8 may be a humoral link between tissue injury and sympathetic hyperalgesia.

The capacity of bradykinin to induce TNFα and to be itself induced by IL-1β reaffirms the importance of bradykinin as a hyperalgesic agent and the therapeutic potential of potent, orally active, antagonists of both types of bradykinin receptor (B$_1$ and B$_2$).

The anti-hyperalgesic effects of cytokines such as IL-4, IL-10 and IL-1ra offers hope that manipulation of the relative balance of proinflammatory and anti-inflammatory cytokines in inflammatory lesions will lead to novel treatments of inflammatory hyperalgesia. Similarly, the discovery of the anti-hyperalgesic effect of LC-1$_{2-26}$ offers another avenue of exploration in the quest for novel anti-hyperalgesic drugs.

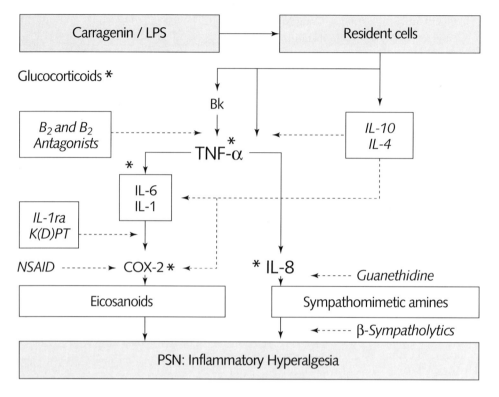

Figure 8
Cytokines and other hyperalgesic agents, and their inhibitors, in inflammatory hyperalgesia.
The postulated roles of cytokines, other hyperalgesic agents and inhibitors of these mediators in inflammatory hyperalgesia. LPS = lipopolysaccharide, BK = bradykinin, B_1 and B_2 =
bradykinin receptors type 1 and type 2, K(D)PT = Lys-D-Pro-Thr, NSAID = non-steroidal anti-
inflammatory drugs, COX-2 = cyclo-oxgenase-2, * = points of therapeutic intervention.

References

1   Henderson B, Poole S (1994) Modulation of cytokine function: therapeutic applications
     In: August JT, Anders MW, Murad F (eds): *Advances in Pharmacology*, Vol 25. Acade-
     mic Press, London, 53–115

2   Ferreira SH, Lorenzetti BB, Bristow AF, Poole S (1988) Interleukin-1beta as a potent
     hyperalgesic agent antagonized by a tripeptide analogue. *Nature* 334: 698–700

3   Schweizer A, Feige U, Fontana A, Muller K, Dinarello CA (1988) Interleukin-1 enhances
     pain reflexes. Mediation through increased prostaglandin E2 levels. *Agents Actions* 25:
     246–251

4   Follenfant RL, Nakamura-Craig M, Henderson B, Higgs GA (1989) Inhibition by neuropeptides of interleukin-1beta-induced, prostaglandin-independent hyperalgesia. *Br J Pharmacol* 98: 41–43

5   Ferreira SH, Lorenzetti BB, Correa FMA (1978) Central and peripheral antialgesic actions of aspirin-like drugs. *Eur J Pharmacol* 53: 39–49

6   McMahon SB, Koltzenburg M (1990) Novel classes of nociceptors: beyond Sherrington. *TINS* 13: 199

7   Ferreira SH (1990) A classification of peripheral analgesics based upon their mode of action. In: Sandler M, Collins GM (eds): *Migraine: Spectrum of ideas*. Oxford University Press, Oxford, 59–72

8   Moncada S, Ferreira SH, Vane JR (1975) Inhibition of prostaglandins biosynthesis as the mechanism of analgesia of aspirin-like drugs in the dog knee joint. *Eur J Pharmacol* 31: 250–260

9   Ferreira SH, Nakamura M, Castro MSA (1978) The hyperalgesic effects of prostacyclin and prostaglandin E2. *Prostaglandins* 16: 31–37

10   Nakamura M, Ferreira SH (1987) A peripheral sympathetic component in inflammatory hyperalgesia. *Eur J Pharmacol* 135: 145–153

11   Duarte IDG, Nakamura M, Ferreira SH (1988) Participation of the sympathetic system in acetic acid-induced writhing in mice. *Brazilian J Med Biol Res* 21: 341–343

12   Coderre TJ, Abbott FV, Melzack R (1984) Effects of peripheral antisympathetic treatments in the tail-flick, formalin and autotomy tests. *Pain* 18: 13-23

13   Wall PD, Gutnick M (1974) Ongoing activity in peripheral nerves: The physiology and pharmacology of impulses originating from a neuroma. *Exp Neurol* 43: 580

14   Ferreira SH (1980) Are macrophages the body's alarm cells? *Agents Actions* 10: 229–230

15   Bernheim HA, Gilbert TM, Stitt JT (1980) Prostaglandin E2 levels in third ventricular cerebrospinal fluid of rabbits during fever and changes in body temperature. *J Physiol* (Lond) 301: 69–78

16   Ferreira SH (1972) Aspirin-like drugs and analgesia. *Nature New Biol* 240: 200–203

17   March CJ, Moseley B, Larsen A, Cerretti DP, Braedt G, Price V, Gillis S, Henney CS, Kronheim SR, Grabstein K et al. (1985) Cloning, sequence and expression of two distinct human interleukin-1 complementary cDNAs. *Nature* 341: 641–646

18   Lumpkin MD (1987) The regulation of ACTH secretion by IL-1. Science 238: 452–454

19   Morstyn G, Burgess AW (1988) Hemopoietic growth factors: a review. *Cancer Res* 48: 5624–5637

20   Stefferl A, Hopkins SJ, Rothwell NJ, Luheshi GN (1996) The role of TNF-alpha in fever: opposing actions of human and murine TNF-alpha and interactions with IL-beta in the rat. *Br J Pharmacol* 118: 1919–1924

21   Garabedian B, Poole S, Allchorne A, Winter J, Woolf CJ (1995) Interleukin-1 beta contributes to the inflammation-induced increase in nerve-growth factor levels and inflammatory hyperalgesia. *Br J Pharmacol* 115: 1265–1275

22 Perkins MN, Kelly D, Davis AJ (1995) Bradykinin B1 and B2 receptor mechanisms and cytokine-induced hyperalgesia in the rat. *Can J Physiol Pharmacol* 73: 832–836

23 Vane JR (1971) Inhibition of prostaglandin synthesis as a mechanism of action of aspirin-like drugs. *Nature* 231: 232–235

24 Dinarello CA (1994) Interleukin-1. In: August JT, Anders MW, Murad F (eds): *Advances in Pharmacology*, Vol 25. Academic Press, London, 21–51

25 Dinarello, CAD (1997) Proinflammatory and anti-inflammatory cytokines as mediators in the pathogenesis of septic shock. *Chest* 112 (6 Suppl): 321S–329S

26 Cunha FQ, Poole S, Lorenzetti BB, Ferreira SH (1991) Interleukin-8 as a mediator of sympathetic pain. *Br J Pharmacol* 104: 765–767

27 Cunha FQ, Poole S, Lorenzetti BB, Ferreira SH (1992) The pivotal role of tumour necrosis factor alpha in the development of inflammatory hyperalgesia. *Br J Pharmacol* 107: 660–664

28 Geng Y, Blanco FJ, Cornelisson M, Lotz M (1995) Regulation of cyclooxygenase-2 expression in normal human articular chondrocytes. *J Immunol* 155: 796–801

29 Burch RM, Connor JR, Axelrod J (1993) Interleukin 1 amplifies receptor-mediated activation of phospholipase A2 in 3T3 fibroblasts. *Proc Natl Acad Sci USA* 85: 6306–6309

30 Dinarello CA, Cannon JG, Wolff SM, Bernheim HA, Beutler B, Cerami A, Figari IS, Palladino MA Jr, O'Connor JV (1986) Tumor necrosis factor (cachectin) is an endogenous pyrogen and induces production of interleukin 1. *J Exp Med* 163: 1433–1450

31 Dinarello CA, Ikejima T, Warner SJ, Orencole SF, Lonnemann G, Cannon JG, Libby P (1987) Interleukin 1 induces interleukin 1. I. Induction of circulating interleukin 1 in rabbits *in vivo* and in human mononuclear cells *in vitro*. *J Immunol* 139: 1902–1910

32 Van Damme J, Opdenakker G, Simpson RJ, Rubira MR, Cayphas S, Vink A, Billiau A, Van Snick J (1987) Identification of the human 26-kD protein, interferon beta 2 (IFN-beta 2), as a B cell hybridoma/plasmacytoma growth factor induced by interleukin 1 and tumor necrosis factor. *J Exp Med* 165: 914–919

33 Streiter RM, Kundel SL, Showell HJ, Remick DG, Phan SH, Ward PA, Marks RM (1989) Endothelial cell gene expression of a neutrophil chemotactic factor by TNF-α, LPS, and IL-1β. *Science* 243: 1467–1469

34 Schindler R, Mancilla J, Endres S, Ghorbani R, Clark SC, Dinarello CA (1990) Correlations and interactions in the production of interleukin-6 (IL-6), IL-1, and tumor necrosis factor (TNF) in human blood mononuclear cells: IL-6 suppresses IL-1 and TNF. *Blood* 75: 40–47

35 Tilg H Trehus E, Atkins MB, Dinarello CA, Mier J.W (1994) Interleukin-6 as an anti-inflammatory cytokine: induction of circulating IL-1 receptor antagonist and soluble tumor necrosis factor receptor p55. *Blood* 83: 113–118

36 Miller AJ, Luheshi GN, Rothwell NJ, Hopkins SJ (1997). Local cytokine induction by LPS in the rat air pouch and its relationship to the febrile response. *Am J Physiol* 272: R857–R861

37 Fong Y, Tracey KJ, Moldawer LL, Hesse DG, Manogue KB, Kenney JS, Lee AT, Kuo GC, Allison AC, Lowry SF et al. (1989) Antibodies to cachectin/tumor necrosis factor

reduce interleukin 1beta and interleukin 6 appearance during lethal bacteremia. *J Exp Med* 170: 1627–1633

38 Gershenwald JE, Fong YM, Fahey TJ, Calvano SE, Chizzonite R, Kilian PL, Lowry SF, Moldawer LL (1990) Interleukin 1 receptor blockade attenuates the host inflammatory response. *Proc Natl Acad Sci USA* 87: 4966–4970

39 Woolf CJ, Allchorne A, Garabedian BS, Poole S (1997) Cytokines, nerve growth factor and inflammatory hyperalgesia: the contribution of tumour necrosis factor alpha. *Br J Pharmacol* 121: 417–424

40 Rothwell NJ (1991). Functions and mechanisms of interleukin 1 in the brain. *Trends Pharmacol Sci* 12: 430–436

41 Armstrong D, Dry RML, Keele CA, Markham JW (1953) Observations on chemical excitants of cutaneous pain in man. *J Physiol* 120: 326–351

42 Lim RKS, Miller DG, Guzman F, Rodgers DW, Rogers RW, Wang SK, Chao PY, Shih TY (1967) Pain and analgesia evaluated by intraperitoneal bradykinin-evoked pain method in man. *Clin Pharmacol Ther* 8: 521–542

43 Sicuteri F, Franciullacci FM, Franchi G, Del Bianco PL (1965) Serotonin-bradykinin potentiation of the pain receptors in man. *Life Sci* 4: 309–316

44 Ferreira SH, Lorenzetti BB, Poole S (1993) Bradykinin initiates cytokine mediated inflammatory hyperalgesia. *Br J Pharmacol* 110: 1227–1231

45 Steranka LR, Dehaas CJ, Vavrek RJ, Stewart JM, Enna SJ, Snyder SH (1987) Antinociceptive effects of bradykinin antagonists. *Eur J Pharmacol* 136: 261–262

46 Costello AH, Hargreaves KM (1989) Suppression of carrageenan hyperalgesia, hyperthermia and edema by a bradykinin antagonist. *Eur J Pharmacol* 171: 259–263

47 Fujiyoshi T, Hayashi I, Oh-ishi S, Kuwashima M, Ilda H, Dozen M, Taniguchi N, Ikeda K, Ohnishi H (1989) Kaolin-induced pain for assessment of analgesic agents. *Agents Actions* 27: 332–334

48 Chau TT, Lewin AC, Walter TL, Carlson RP, Weichman BM (1991) Evidence for a role of bradykinin in experimental pain models. *Agents Actions* 34: 235–238

49 Beresford IJM, Birch PJ (1992) Antinociceptive activity of the bradykinin antagonist HOE 140 in rat and mouse. *Br J Pharmacol* 105 (suppl): 1P–314P

50 Tiffany CW, Burch RM (1989) Bradykinin stimulates tumour necrosis factor and interleukin-1 release from macrophages. *FEBS Lett* 247: 189–192

51 Davis AJ, Perkins MN (1994) The involvement of bradykinin B1 and B2 receptor mechanisms in cytokine-induced mechanical hyperalgesia in the rat. *Br J Pharmacol* 113: 63–68

52 Dray A, Perkins M (1993) Bradykinin and inflammatory pain. *Trends Neurosci* 16: 99–104

53 Steranka LR, Manning DC, Dehass CJ (1988) Bradykinin as pain mediator: receptors are localized to sensory neurons and antagonists have analgesic actions. *Proc Natl Acad Sci USA* 85: 3245–3249

54 Nagy I, Pabla R, Matesz C, Dray A, Woolf CJ, Urban L (1993) Cobalt uptake enables

identification of capsaicin- and bradykinin-sensitive subpopulations of rat dorsal root ganglion cells *in vitro*. *Neuroscience* 56: 241–246

55 Davis CL, Naeem S, Phagoo SB, Campbell EA, Urban L, Burgess GM (1996) B1 bradykinin receptors and sensory neurones. *Br J Pharmacol* 118:1469–1476

56 Rothschild AM, Gascon LA (1966) Sulphuric esters of polysaccharides as activators of a bradykinin-forming system in plasma. *Nature* 212: 1364

57 Damas J, Remacle-Volon G (1992) Influence of a long-acting bradykinin antagonist, Hoe 140, on some acute inflammatory reactions in the rat. *Eur J Pharmacol* 211: 81–86

58 Vannier E, Miller LC, Dinarello CA (1992) Co-ordinated anti-inflammatory effects of interleukin-4: Interleukin-4 suppresses interleukin-1 production but up-regulates gene expression and synthesis of interleukin-1 receptor antagonist. *Proc Natl Acad Sci USA* 89: 4076–4080

59 Fenton MJ, Buras JA, Donelly RP (1992) IL-4 reciprocally regulates IL-1 and IL-1 receptor antagonist expression in human monocytes. *J Immunol* 149: 1283–1288

60 Wright SD, Ramos RA, Tobias PS, Ulevitch RJ, Mathison JC (1990). CD14, a receptor for complexes of lipopolysaccharide (LPS) and LPS binding protein. *Science* 249: 1431–1433

61 Lauener RP, Goyert SM, Geha RS, Vercelli D (1990) Interleukin-4 down-regulates the expression of CD14 in normal human monocytes. *Eur J Immunol* 20: 2375–2381

62 Fiorentino DF, Bond MW, Mosmann TR (1989) Two types of mouse helper T cell IV. Th2 clones secrete a factor that inhibits cytokine production by Th1 clones. *J Exp Med* 170: 2081–2095

63 Zlotnik A, Moore KW (1991) Interleukin-10. *Cytokine* 3: 366–371

64 Howard M, O'Garra A (1992) Biological properties of IL-10. *Immunol Today* 13: 198–200

65 De Waal Malefyt R, Haanen J, Spits H, Roncarolo MG, Tevelde A, Figdor C, Johnson K, Kastelein R, Yssel H, Devries J (1991) Interleukin-10 (IL-10) and viral IL-10 strongly reduce antigen-specific human T cell proliferation by diminishing the antigen-presenting capacity of monocytes via downregulation of class II major histocompatibility complex expression. *J Exp Med* 174: 915–925

66 Fiorentino DF, Zlotnik A, Mossmann TR, Howard M, O'Garra A (1991) IL-10 inhibits cytokine production by activated macrophages. *J Immunol* 147: 3815–3822

67 De Waal Malefyt R, Abrams J, Bennett B, Figdor CG, Devries JE (1991) Interleukin-10 (IL-10) inhibits cytokine synthesis by human monocytes: an autoregulatory role of IL-10 produced by monocytes. *J Exp Med* 174: 1209–1220

68 Bogdan C, Vodovotz Y, NathanC (1991) Macrophage deactivation by interleukin-10. *J Exp Med* 174: 1549–1555

69 Oswald IP, Wynn TA, Sher A, James,SL (1992) Interleukin-10 inhibits macrophage microbicidal activity by blocking the endogenous production of tumor necrosis factor alpha required as a costimulatory factor for interferon gamma-induced activation. *Proc Natl Acad Sci USA* 89: 8676–8680

70 Howard M, O'Garra A, Ishida H, De Waal Malefyt R de Vries J (1992) Biological properties of interleukin 10. *J Clin Immunol* 12: 239–247

71 Poole S, Cunha FQ, Selkirk S, Lorenzetti BB, Ferreira SH (1995) Cytokine-mediated inflammatory hyperalgesia limited by interleukin-10. *Br J Pharmacol* 115: 684–688

72 Mertz PM, Dewitt DL, Stelter-Stevenson G, Wahl LM (1994) Interleukin 10 suppression of monocyte prostaglandin H Synthase-2. *J Biol Chem* 269: 21322–21329

73 Flower RJ, Rothwell NJ (1994) Lipocortin-1: cellular mechanisms and clinical relevance. *TiPS* 15: 71–76

74 Relton JK, Strijbos PJ, O'Shaughnessy CT, Carey F, Forder RA, Tilders FJ, Rothwell NJ (1991) Lipocortin-1 is an endogenous inhibitor of ischaemic damage in the rat brain. *J Exp Med* 174: 305–310

75 Perretti M, Ahluwalia A, Harris JG, Harris HJ, Wheller SK, Flower RJ (1996) Acute inflammatory response in the mouse: exacerbation by immunoneutralization of lipocortin-1. *Br J Pharmacol* 117: 1145–1154

76 Perretti M, Ahluwalia A, Harris JG, Goulding NJ, Flower RJ (1993) Lipocortin-1 fragments inhibit neutrophil-dependent edema in the mouse. *J Immunol* 151: 4306–4314

77 Ferreira SH, Cunha FQ, Lorenzetti, B.B., Michelin MA, Perretti M, Flower RJ, Poole S (1997) Role of lipocortin-1 in the analgesic actions of glucocorticoids. *Br J Pharmacol* 121: 883–888

78 Blackwell, GJ, Carnuccio, R, Dirosa, M, Flower, RJ, Parente, L, Perisco, P (1980) Macrocortin: a polypeptide causing the anti-phospholipase effect of glucocorticoid drugs. *Nature* 287: 147–149

79 Hirata F, Schiffmann E, Venkatasubamanian K, Salomon D, Axelrod J (1980) A phospholipase A2 inhibitory protein in rabbit neutrophils induced by glucocorticoids. *Proc Natl Acad Sci USA* 77: 2533–2536

80 Waage A, Bakke O (1988) Glucocorticoids suppress the production of tumour necrosis factor by lipopolysaccharide-stimulated human monocytes. *Immunology* 63: 299–302

81 Lew W, Oppenheim JJ, Matsushima K (1988) Analysis of the suppression of IL-1 alpha and IL-1 beta production in human peripheral blood mononuclear adherent cells by a glucocorticoid hormone. *J Immunol* 140: 1895–1902

82 Barton BE, Jakaway JP, Smith SR, Siegel MI (1991) Cytokine inhibition by a novel steroid, mometasone furoate. *Immunopharmacol Immunotoxicol* 13: 251–261

83 Seitz M, Dewald B, Gerber N, Baggiolini M (1991) Enhanced production of neutrophil-activating peptide-1 interleukin-8 in rheumatoid arthritis. *J Clin Invest* 87: 463–469

84 Auphan N, Didonato JA, Rosette C, Helmberg A, Karin M (1995). Immunosuppression by glucocorticoids: inhibition of NF-κB activity through induction of Iκ synthesis. *Science* 270: 286–290

85 Scheinman RI, Gogswell PC, Lofquist AK, Baldwin Jr AS (1995) Role of transcriptional activation of 1κBα in mediation of immunosuppression by glucocorticoids. *Science* 270: 283–286

86 Sterling EA, Barthelmäs R, Pfeuffer I, Schenk B, Zarius S, Swoboda R, Mercurio F, Karin

M (1989) Ubiquitous and lymphocyte-specific factors are involved in the induction of the mouse interleukin-2 gene in T lymphocytes. *EMBO J* 8: 465–473

87 Park J-H, Kaushansky K, Levitt L (1993) Transcriptional regulation of interleukin-3 in primary human lymphocytes. *J Biol Chem* 268: 6299–6308

88 Cockerill PN, Shannon MF, Bert AG, Ryan GR, Vadas MA (1993) The granulocyte-macrophage colony stimulating factor/interleukin-3 locus is regulated by an inducible cyclosporin A-sensitive enhancer. *Proc Natl Acad Sci USA* 90: 2466–2470

89 Stein B, Baldwin AS, Ballard DW, Greene WC, Angel P, Herrlich P (1993) Cross-coupling of the NF-κB p65 and Fos-Jun transcription factors produces potentiated biological function. *EMBO J* 12: 3879–3891

90 Flower RJ, Blackwell GJ (1979) Anti-inflammatory steroids induce biosynthesis of a phospholipase A2 inhibitor which prevents prostaglandin generation. *Nature* 278 (5703): 456–459

91 Lorenzetti BB, Ferreira SH (1985) Mode of analgesic action of dipyrone: direct antagonism of inflammatory hyperalgesia. *Eur J Pharmacol* 114: 375–381

92 Katsuki H, Nakai S, Hirai Y, Akaji K, Kiso Y, Satoh M (1990) Interleukin-1 beta inhibits long-term potentiation in the CA3 region of mouse hippocampal slices. *Eur J Pharmacol* 181: 323–326

93 Hua XY, Chen P, Fox A, Myers RR (1996) Involvement of cytokines in lipopolysaccharide-induced facilitation of CGRP release from capsaicin-sensitive nerves in the trachea: studies with interleukin-1beta and tumor necrosis factor-alpha. *J Neurosci* 16: 4742–4748

94 Davis AK, Perkins MN (1996) desArg9BK-induced mechanical hyperalgesia and analgesia in the rat: involvement of IL-1, prostaglandins and peripheral opioids. *Br J Pharmacol Proceedings* (Suppl) Dec 1996, 74P

95 Marceau F, Petitclerc E, Deblois D, Pradelles, Poubell PE (1991) Human interleukin-1 induces a rapid relaxation of the rabbit isolated mesenteric artery. *Br J Pharmacol* 103: 1367–1372

96 Poole S, Bristow AF, Lorenzetti BB, Gaines Das RE, Smith TW, Ferreira SH, (1992). Peripheral analgesic activities of peptides related to alpha-MSH and interleukin-1 beta 193-195. *Br J Pharmacol* 106: 489–492

97 Richards DB, Lipton JM (1984) Effect of alpha-MSH 11-13 (lysine-proline-valine) on fever in the rabbit. *Peptides* 5: 815–817

98 Dinarello CA (1984) Interleukin-1. *Rev Infect Dis* 6: 51–95

99 Hiltz ME, Lipton JM (1989) Anti-inflammatory activity of a COOH-terminal fragment of the neuropeptide α-MSH. *Res Commun* 3: 2282–2284

100 Hiltz ME, Lipton JM (1990) Alpha-MSH peptides inhibit acute inflammation and contact sensitivity. *Peptides* 11: 979–982

101 Deeter LB, Martin LW, Lipton JM (1989) Antipyretic properties of centrally administered alpha-MSH fragments in the rabbit. *Peptides* 9: 1285–1288

102 Safieh-Garabedian B, Kanaan SA, Jalakhian RH, Poole S, Jabbur SJ, Saade NE (1997)

Hyperalgesia induced by low doses of thymulin injections: possible involvement of prostaglandin E2. *J Neuroimmunol* 1997 73: 162–168

103 Walker JM, Akil H, Watson SJ (1980) Evidence for homologous actions of pro-opio-cortin products. *Science* 210: 1247–1249

104 Ohkubo T, Shibata M, Takahashi H, Naruse S (1985) Naloxone prevents the analgesic action of alpha-MSH in mice. *Experientia* 41: 627–628

105 Oluyomi AO, Poole S, Smith TW, Hart SL (1994) Antinociceptive activity of peptides related to interleukin-1 beta-(193-195), Lys-Pro-Thr. *Eur J Pharmacol* 1994 258: 131–138

106 Lyson K, Ceriani G, Takashima A, Catania A, Lipton JM (1994) Binding of anti-inflammatory alpha-melanocyte-stimulating-hormone peptides and proinflammatory cytokines to receptors on melanoma cells. *Neuroimmunomodulation* 1994: 121–126

Cytokine-nerve growth factor interactions in inflammatory hyperalgesia

Stephen Poole[1] and Clifford J. Woolf[2]

[1]Division of Endocrinology, National Institute for Biological Standards and Control, Blanche Lane, South Mimms, Potters Bar, Herts EN6 3QG, UK; [2]Neural Plasticity Research Group, Dept of Anesthesia, Massachusetts General Hospital and Harvard Medical School, 149 13th Street, Room 4309, Charlestown, MA 02129, USA

General concepts

Plasticity of the primary sensory neuron (PSN)

Primary sensory neurons interface between the external environment and the central nervous system. To detect and transfer to the CNS information describing the stimuli that impinge upon the body, the PSN have highly specialized adaptations. These include the expression of a broad number of ion channels, receptors, neurotransmitters and neuromodulators, together with the establishment of highly ordered patterns of innervation of the peripheral target and central neurons.

A substantial body of data has been gathered regarding the intrinsic and extrinsic factors that cause a neural crest progenitor cell to become a mature, specialized sensory neuron. Obviously neurotrophins play a major role, both in terms of differentiation and survival, that manifests itself during the establishment of neuron-target interactions during development. Less attention has been paid to the possibility that the phenotype of mature, differentiated neurons in the adult is not fixed and that phenotypic modification constitutes an important element in the alteration of sensory neuron function in different pathological conditions [1].

The first evidence to suggest phenotypic modification of adult PSN came from studies on the consequences of disrupting contact of the neuron with its target by cutting the peripheral axon (these studies are reviewed in [2]). Peripheral axotomy led to a characteristic set of changes, including the down-regulation of a number of neuropeptides, such as substance P (SP) and calcitonin gene related peptide (CGRP), and the expression of other neuropeptides, such as vasoactive intestinal polypeptide (VIP), neuropeptide Y (NPY) and galanin. Many, but not all, of these chemical changes can be prevented by administration of neurotrophins [3], and this has been interpreted as evidence for a role for target-produced growth factors in maintaining the normal phenotype of the PSN.

Until recently the consequences of the converse situation were not considered. That is, the consequences of exposing the PSN to increased concentrations of neurotrophins, e.g. nerve growth factor (NGF), in their target tissue, and whether this leads to a change in phenotype and whether such a change modifies their function. This chapter surveys evidence showing that this is indeed the case for inflammation and inflammatory pain hypersensitivity.

Interactions of NGF with inflammatory mediators other than cytokines

Inflammation is associated with a complex pattern of local and systemic changes, including inflammatory cell migration, cytokine release, oedema, erythema, release of acute phase proteins, fever, pain and hyperalgesia. The sequence of events that leads to the sensory changes at the site of the inflammation and in the surrounding tissue are, as yet, poorly understood, although changes both in the transduction sensitivity of the high threshold nociceptors and in the excitability in the CNS secondary to the activation of chemosensitive nociceptors by inflammatory mediators are involved [4, 5]. The mediators responsible include K^+, H^+, ATP, arachidonic acid derivatives, cytokines, bradykinin, tachykinins, serotonin and histamine, operating together in a synergistic way [4, 5] to increase transduction sensitivity of high threshold nociceptors by phosphorylating sodium channels [6]. Recently it has become apparent that the neurotrophin nerve growth factor (NGF) also plays a major role in the production of inflammatory hyperalgesia [7, 8].

The role of NGF in the development and maintenance of peripheral sympathetic and nociceptive sensory neurons is well established [9–11]. NGF is produced in the peripheral target, binds to a high affinity receptor tyrosine kinase, *trkA*, on the neuron and, after internalization, is retrogradely transported to the cell body where, by activation of second messenger signals and changes in transcription factor expression, it controls the survival, growth and phenotype of immature neurons [10, 12–15]. In addition to this specific neurotrophic action during development, a constant supply of NGF from the periphery may be important for the maintenance of normal phenotype in *trkA* receptor expressing nociceptive adult primary sensory neurons [16]. Removal of NGF results in a down-regulation of several transmitters and proteins [17–19] whereas an excess results in abnormal sensitivity [20]. Systemic NGF administration, for example, induces thermal and mechanical hyperalgesia in neonatal and adult rats [21] and intraplantar (i.pl.) NGF produces localized thermal hyperalgesia in adult rats [7].

During inflammation concentrations of NGF are increased in 'inflammatory cells' (mast cells), inflammatory exudates (ascites/synovial fluid), inflamed skin, and in the nerves innervating inflamed tissue [7, 22–25]. Also, the hyperalgesia associated with the inflammation resulting from injection of Complete Freund's adjuvant (CFA) was markedly attenuated following systemic administration of a specific sheep anti-NGF antiserum [7] suggesting that NGF contributes directly or indirectly to changes in inflammatory sensitivity. The indirect effects of NGF may result from its cytokine-like actions, including stimulation of growth and differentiation of human B lymphocytes [5, 26, 27], the release of inflammatory mediators from lymphocytes and basophils [28, 29] and degranulation of mast cells [30-33]. Direct effects could be either due to a *trkA* receptor tyrosine kinase-mediated phosphorylation at the nociceptor terminal, increasing transduction sensitivity, or a consequence of a change in the expression of transmitter/neuromodulators such as SP and CGRP in the cell body [7, 16], amplifying the central actions of the nociceptor in the spinal cord [8]. SP and CGRP are present in C-fibres and coexist in up to 20% of dorsal root ganglion (DRG) neurons [34]. Expression of both peptides is modulated by NGF in adult sensory neuron cultures [16, 18], and both are upregulated during inflammation [7, 24, 35–37]. Anti-NGF prevents the inflammatory increase in the peptides [7, 24]. These neuropeptides are released from the central terminals of C-fibres and have excitatory effects on dorsal horn neurons controlling the gain of nociceptive transmission [38]. Whether the role of NGF in inflammatory hyperalgesia is related to changes in neuropeptide concentrations in sensory neurons is not known.

Experimental inflammatory hypersensitivity

A number of the studies described below involved inflammation induced by the administration of CFA (100 μl) into the plantar surface of the left hind-paw (intraplantar, i.pl.) under anaesthesia. The CFA produced an area of localized erythema and oedema, responses which did not disturb weight gain, grooming, the sleep-wake cycle or social interactions. Mechanical hyperalgesia was assessed using a set of Von Frey hairs (4.1 to 72 g). The minimum force required to elicit a reproducible flexor withdrawal reflex on each of 3 applications of the Von Frey hairs to the dorsal surface of the toes was measured [7, 39]. Thermal hypersensitivity was assessed using the hot-plate technique, measuring the time for foot withdrawal on contact with a metal plate at 50° C. Oedema was scored on a scale from 0 (no swelling) to 5 (swelling on plantar and dorsal surface of hind-paw and all toes).

Behavioural measurements were made immediately before and at intervals after injection (i.pl.) of CFA (or saline). The L4 dorsal root ganglion (DRG) and entire hind-paw skin, ipsilateral and contralateral to the inflammation, were removed for assay of inflammatory mediators. Anti-hyperalgesic agents (inhibitors, antagonists and antibodies) were injected (in 100 μl, unless indicated otherwise) via the routes and at the time intervals specified below. Dexamethasone (120 mg kg^{-1}) was given intramuscularly (i.m.), once daily (lower dose) or three times daily (higher dose), before and after CFA. Indomethacin (2 or 4 mg kg^{-1}) was given intraperitoneally (i.p.), lower dose or higher dose, once daily, before and after CFA.

NGF as a mediator of inflammatory hyperalgesia

There is a growing body of data to suggests that inflammation is accompanied by a marked increase in (NGF) production and that NGF is a principal mediator of inflammatory hyperalgesia. NGF-mediated alteration of the chemical phenotype of the PSN appears to be an essential component of the sensory alterations that occur subsequent to inflammation and which manifests as inflammatory hyperalgesia [1].

NGF and hyperalgesia

That NGF may have the capacity in the adult to increase sensitivity to noxious stimuli, that is to produce hyperalgesia, first emerged from studies in which large doses of systemically administered NGF evoked both thermal and mechanical hyperalgesia in rats [21]. Similar findings were reported in mice [40] and in man [41]. Local injections of NGF also evoked sensitivity changes in rats [7] and in man [41]. Intraplantar (i.pl.) injections of NGF (2 ng to 2 mg), resulted in a relatively short-lived increase in mechanical and thermal hypersensitivity (Fig. 1A) which, except at the highest dose, was over within 24 h. The onset of the hypersensitivity change was too early for a transcription-related change as the NGF would have required retrograde transport from the site of injection to the cell bodies of the sensory neurons in the lumbar dorsal root ganglia which, at the maximal fast axonal transport rate, would have taken ~5–6 h. Following transcription, any novel protein would then have required transport to the peripheral or central terminal before it could effect a change in function. It is likely, therefore, that the immediate sensitivity changes produced by NGF were mediated peripherally.

Although the sensitivity changes produced by NGF (200 ng) were transient, the NGF caused alterations in the phenotype of sensory neurons innervating the site of the NGF administration. The concentrations of the neuropeptides SP and CGRP were elevated in the sciatic nerve post NGF injection [7, 24] and there was a substantial increase in the number of dorsal root ganglion cells staining positive for preprotachykinin A and CGRP mRNA [42] (Fig. 1B). These data confirmed the suggestion that the concentration of SP in adult dorsal root ganglion cells is controlled by the concentration of NGF in the target [18], although cultured cells are necessarily axotomized and might not react in the same way as intact neurons *in vivo*.

Inflammation and NGF

A number of cell types can express NGF [25, 43, 44] and increased concentrations of NGF have been described in the distal stumps of degenerated nerves [45], in inflammatory exudates (Weskamp and Otten, 1987 [22]), in the synovium of inflamed joints [46], in skin wounds [47], and after adjuvant inflammation [7]. Inflammation evoked by local injection of CFA into one hind-paw resulted in a sig-

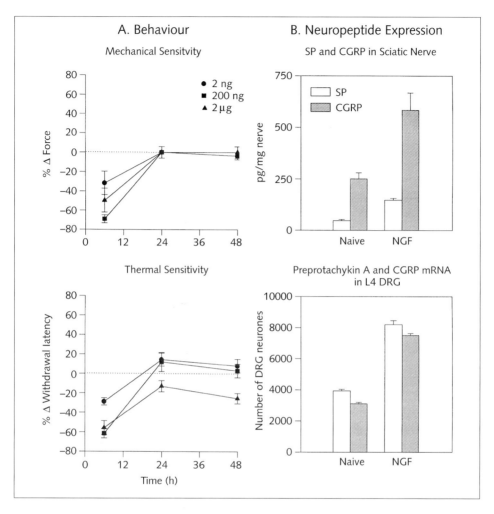

Figure 1

Effects of NGF on thermal and mechanical sensitivity and on the production of SP and CGRP. (A) Effects of NGF (200 ng, i.pl.) on thermal and mechanical sensitivity in rats. Mechanical sensitivity (upper panel) was measured by the change in threshold for eliciting a flexion withdrawal reflex using Von Frey hairs. Thermal sensitivity (lower panel) was measured by the change in reaction time in a hot-plate test (50° C). Data have been normalised to the pre-injection concentrations (means ± s.e.m., n = 5). The symbols represent doses of NGF: circles = 2 ng, squares = 200 ng, triangles = 2 μg. Panel (B) Effect of NGF (200 ng, i.pl.) on the expression of SP (open columns) and CGRP (hatched columns) in sciatic nerves innervating the injected paws, measured by immunoassay (upper panel) and by changes in the number of L4 dorsal root ganglion (DRG) cells expressing preprotachykinin A or CGRP (measured by non-isotopic in situ *hybridization, lower panel). Reproduced with permission from [1].*

nificant increase in NGF concentrations in the inflamed skin and the sciatic nerve innervating the site of the inflammation [1, 7]. The latter indicates that the increased local production of NGF results in retrograde transport of the neurotrophin [48], presumably in *trkA*-expressing sensory fibres [49].

The increase in NGF concentrations contributes significantly to inflammatory hypersensitivity since the administration of a neutralizing sheep anti-NGF serum prior to the induction of adjuvant inflammation prevented the establishment of mechanical and thermal hypersensitivity (Fig. 2A) [7]. This finding has been substantiated in other studies [8], including one that utilised the novel approach of a *trkA*-IgG fusion protein to compete for the NGF [50].

It is possible that NGF may be only an early mediator in the production of inflammation hypersensitivity. To test this hypothesis, sheep anti-NGF serum was administered after the induction of inflammation, at a time when the hypersensitivity was fully developed. In these circumstances, thermal hypersensitivity was substantially reduced 1 h after injecting the anti-serum. This suggests that an ongoing supply of NGF in the periphery contributes to the maintenance of the thermal hyperalgesia. Since the reversal took place so quickly, the NGF must have been acting (either directly or indirectly) on the peripheral terminals, to alter transduction sensitivity, that is, NGF appears to contribute to the peripheral sensitization of high threshold thermoreceptors, in a manner that has a short half-life and that requires, therefore, a continuous supply of NGF.

Mechanical hypersensitivity, induced by adjuvant inflammation, was not immediately reversed by sheep anti-NGF serum, unlike thermal sensitivity (Fig. 2B). Rather, a reduction in mechanical sensitivity only manifested itself 24 h after the administration of the anti-NGF serum and became more pronounced at 36 h and especially at 48 h [1, 7]. The delay before an effect of removing peripheral NGF could be detected may well reflect the time required for retrograde transport to the

Figure 2
Effect of anti-NGF serum on CFA-induced mechanical sensitivity and thermosensitivity.
(A) CFA-induced (100 µl, i.pl., squares) inflammation in the hind-paws produces a rapid and marked increases in mechanical sensitivity (left hand panel) and thermosensitivity (right hand panel). This was almost completely prevented by systemic pre-treatment with a specific neutralizing sheep-anti-NGF serum (5 µl g⁻¹, 1 h before the CFA, circles). (B) When inflammatory hypersensitivity in response to CFA was well established, administration of the anti-NGF serum (circles) at day 5 resulted, within 1 h, in a marked reduction in thermal hypersensitivity (right hand panel). Mechanical hypersensitivity (left hand panel) was decreased only at 24–48 h after administration of the anti-NGF serum. This delay is consistent with an interruption of NGF-mediated changes in transcription in the DRG). Reproduced with permission from [1].

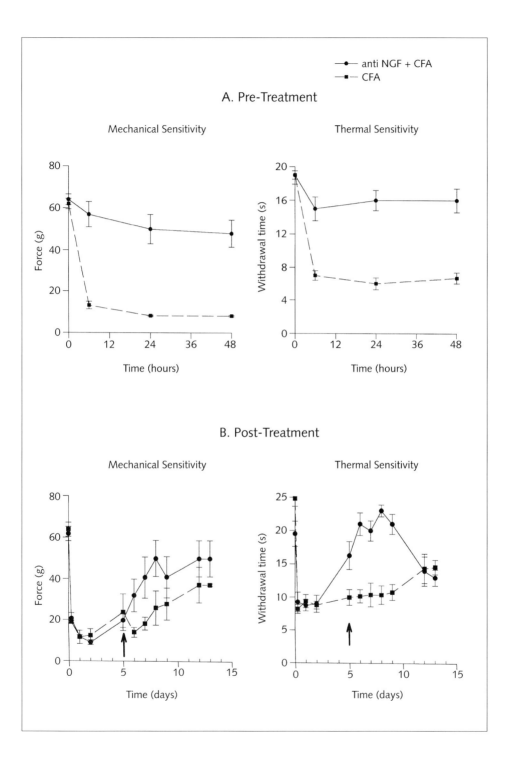

DRG, signal transduction, altered transcription and translation and protein/peptide transport [1].

Phenotypic modifications after inflammation

Acute inflammation leads to changes in the concentrations of neuropeptides SP and CGRP in primary sensory neurones [7, 24, 35, 42, 51]. The extent to which the increases in concentrations of peptides is due to an increased production by cells which usually produce these peptides or to the production by cells which normally do not produce the peptides has not been fully resolved. It is clear that the number of DRG cells positive for preprotachykinin A and CGRP mRNA increased more than two-fold following the induction of adjuvant-induced inflammation in the hind-paw (Fig. 3). Since approximately 20% of lumbar DRG cells are usually positive for SP (using immunohistochemical and *in situ* techniques), and since the total number of L4 DRG neurons is 16–18,000, many more neurons innervating the inflamed paw were expressing mRNA for preprotachykinin A than in the absence of inflammation. Whether all these cells express the peptide (SP) is not known but there is a significant increase in the number of myelinated afferents which are positive for SP after inflammation. This indicates that there is a change in phenotype after inflammation. The fact that anti-NGF administration effectively prevented inflammation-induced changes in mRNA and peptide (Fig. 3) shows that NGF is involved.

In addition to changes in neuropeptides, CFA-induced inflammation also affected concentrations of the growth-associated protein GAP-43 [42]. The time course of the increase in GAP-43 mRNA and preprotachykinin A mRNA were very similar and both were restricted to the dorsal root ganglion innervating the inflamed tissue (Fig. 3B). However, although mRNA for both GAP-43 and preprotachykinin A was increased in an NGF-dependent fashion following inflammation, only mRNA for preprotachykinin A was increased following the administration of NGF [42]. This shows that NGF administration does not model the inflammatory state and that while NGF is necessary it is not sufficient in itself to cause all the phenotypic changes that occur in adjuvant inflammation.

Cytokine-NGF interactions in inflammatory hyperalgesia

Interleukin-1β contributes to inflammation-induced increases in NGF concentrations and inflammatory hyperalgesia

IL-1β induces NGF

An important question is what controls the production of NGF during inflammation. An obvious candidate was interleukin-1β (IL-1β), a cytokine involved in a wide

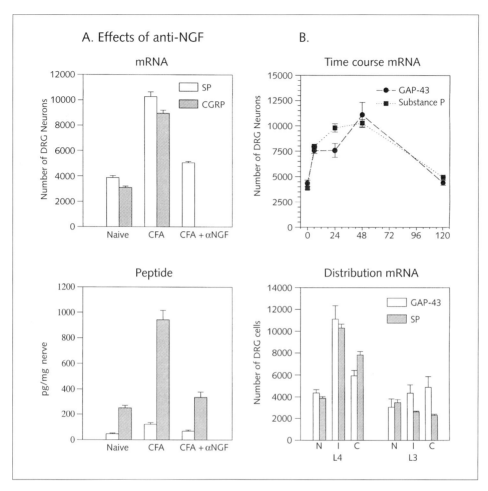

Figure 3
Phenotypic changes in the DRG and sciatic nerve, 48 h after CFA-induced inflammation.
(A) CFA-induced (100 µl, i.pl.) changes in the expression of preprotachykinin A (open columns) and CGRP (hatched columns) mRNA in the DRG (lower panel) and concentrations of peptides (open columns = SP; hatched columns = CGRP) in the sciatic nerve (bottom panel), 48 h after CFA, and prevention of the increases by sheep anti-NGF serum (5 µl g⁻¹, 1 h before the CFA,). (CGRP mRNA + anti-NGF not tested). (B) Time course of changes in the number of DRG neurones expressing preprotachykinin A and GAP-43 mRNA after induction of adjuvant inflammation in one hind-paw (upper panel). The lower panels show that the increase in expression is limited to that ganglion (L4) innervating the inflamed site. The adjacent ganglion (L3) shows no change. N = naive, I = ipsilateral to inflammation, C = contralateral hind-paw. Open columns = SP; hatched columns = GAP-43; squares represent SP; circles represent GAP-43. Reproduced with permission from [1].

variety of inflammatory responses [52–54]. Numerous cell types produce IL-1β, including blood monocytes, tissue macrophages, blood neutrophils, endothelial cells, smooth muscle cells, fibroblasts, dermal dendritic cells, keratinocytes, and T and B lymphocytes [53, 55]. IL-1β concentrations are raised during inflammation [56, 57], and its administration by various routes evokes hyperalgesia [58–62]. Systemic IL-1β evoked a thermal hyperalgesia and mediated the hyperalgesic response to bacterial endotoxin (lipopolysaccharide, LPS) [62]. IL-1β injection into hind-paws (i.pl.) evoked a dose-dependent increase in sensitivity to low intensity mechanical pressure [58] and thermal hyperalgesia [51, 63] but no change in the threshold for eliciting a flexion withdrawal reflex [51]. This difference between the two models of mechanical hyperalgesia probably relates to the different nature of the tests and endpoints used. IL-1β can induce NGF production in a number of cell types [43, 45, 64–67] and the development of specific immunoassays (ELISAs) for NGF and IL-1β, permitted a putative role for IL-1β in NGF production in inflammatory lesions to be investigated [51].

Roles for NGF and IL-1β in CFA-induced inflammatory hyperalgesia

Acute inflammation in hind-paws caused by CFA injection (i.pl.) resulted in significant increases in NGF (Fig. 4) and IL-1β (Fig. 5) concentrations in the inflamed tissue, with a much greater relative change in the latter. The inflammation also resulted in an elevation in the concentrations of neuropeptides (Fig. 6) in the primary sensory neurons innervating the inflamed hind-limb and in substantial thermal and mechanical (Fig. 7) hyperalgesia [51].

Figure 4

Effects of indomethacin and dexamethasone on CFA-induced increases in concentrations of NGF.

The inflammation induced by intraplantar CFA injection (100 μl, i.pl.) caused a significant increase in NGF concentrations, measured 48 h after CFA injection, in ipsilateral hind-paws (open columns) compared with naïve animals (hatched columns). The lower dose dexamethasone (Dex) treatment (120 μg kg^{-1}, daily) had no significant effect on NGF concentration but the higher dose regimen (120 μg kg^{-1}, 8 hourly) prevented the increases (upper panel). The lower dose of indomethacin (Ind, 2 mg kg^{-1}, daily) had no significant effect on NGF concentrations in the ipsilateral hind-paw, but the higher dose (4 mg kg^{-1}, daily) prevented the CFA-induced increases (lower panel). Data are mean ± s.e.m., n = 5, [a]p < 0.05; [a]p < 0.01 and [a**]p < 0.001 vs naive; [b]p < 0.05; [b**]p < 0.001 low vs high doses; [c]p < 0.05, [c*]p < 0.01 vs CFA; [d]p < 0.01; [d**]p < 0.001 ipsilateral vs contralateral. Reproduced with permission from [51].*

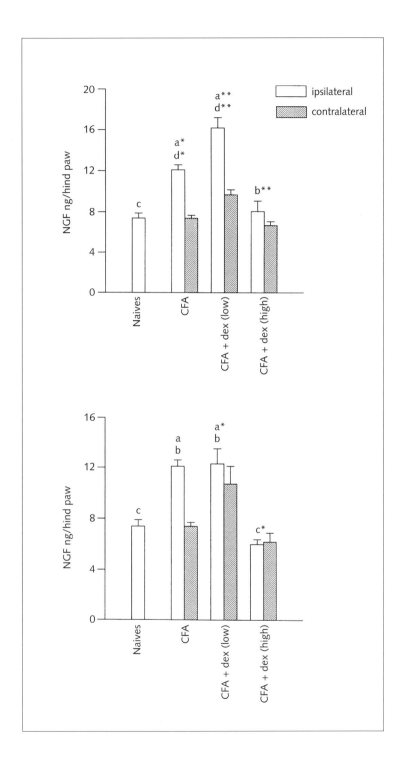

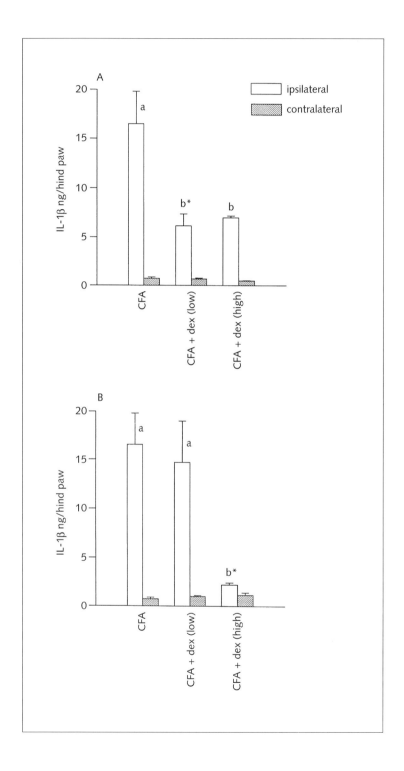

Antagonism of IL-1β action during the establishment of CFA inflammation reduced acute mechanical hyperalgesia but had a smaller effect on established inflammatory hyperalgesia (Fig. 7) [51]. The mechanism of IL-1β-induced changes in sensitivity has been variously argued to be mediated via PG production [58,68, 69], independently of PG-production [62, 70], via the induction of bradykinin B_1 receptors [71], or as a result of a direct activation of nociceptors [61]. Another possibility is that IL-1β produced its effects by upregulating an active intermediary such as NGF. IL-1β caused NGF production by cultured fibroblasts [43, 65, 66] and evoked hyperalgesia when administered either systemically [20] or locally [7]. Also, IL-1β evoked increases in NGF concentrations in the skin and neutralisation of the action of NGF inhibited the hyperalgesic actions of IL-1β (Fig. 8) [51]. IL-1β regulated SP concentrations in sympathetic ganglion cells [72] through the induction of a neuropoietic cytokine, leukaemia inhibitory factor (LIF) [73]. IL-1β may have altered neuropeptide expression in primary sensory neurons secondary to an increase in NGF concentrations since NGF has well known actions on the regulation of both SP and CGRP in adult DRG neurons [7, 16, 18]. Certainly anti-NGF antibodies inhibited the increase in concentrations of SP and CGRP associated with CFA-induced inflammation [7, 24], even though they did not inhibit upregulation of IL-1β [51].

NGF concentrations are substantially increased during inflammation [7, 22–24]. The specific signalling mechanisms and cell types responsible are not known, although IL-1β appears to have a major role in increasing NGF production in that the IL-1 receptor antagonist (IL-1ra) attenuated the increase in NGF concentrations subsequent to injection of CFA (Fig. 7) and IL-1β (Fig. 8). A number of other growth factors/inflammatory mediators may also be involved. Platelet derived growth factor (PDGF), acidic and basic fibroblast growth factor (α and βFGF),

Figure 5
Effects of indomethacin and dexamethasone on CFA-induced increases in concentrations of IL-1β.
The inflammation induced by CFA (100 μl, i.pl.) caused a significant increase in IL-1β concentrations in ipsilateral paws (open columns) at 48 h post CFA injection compared with the contralateral hind-paws (hatched columns). Both the lower (120 μg/kg^{-1}, 8 hourly) and higher (120 μg/kg^{-1}, 8 hourly) dose dexamethasone treatments significantly reduced IL-1β concentrations in ipsilateral hind-paws (A). The lower dose indomethacin (Ind, 2 mg kg^{-1}, daily) had no significant effect on IL-1β concentrations but the higher dose (4 mg kg^{-1}, daily) significantly reduced concentrations of this cytokine in ipsilateral paws (B). Data are mean ± s.e.m., n = 5 , $^{a**}p < 0.001$ ipsilateral vs contralateral; $^{b}p < 0.05$; $^{b*}p < 0.01$ vs ipsilateral CFA. Reproduced with permission from [51].

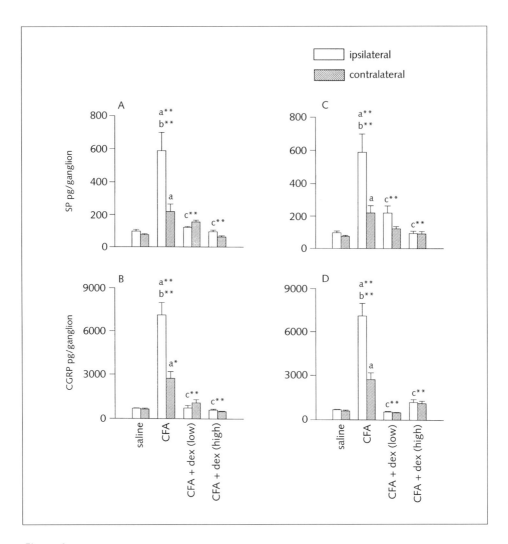

Figure 6

Effect of indomethacin and dexamethasone on CFA-induced increases in concentrations of SP and CGRP in the ipsilateral L4 DRG.

CFA-induced inflammation caused significant increases in SP (A and C) and CGRP (lower panels) concentrations in the ipsilateral L4 DRG (open columns), measured at 48 h, compared with the contralateral side (hatched columns) or with animals receiving vehicle instead of CFA. Both the lower dose and the higher dose dexamethasone (Dex, left hand columns) and indomethacin (Ind) treatments (right hand columns) prevented CFA-induced increases in SP and CGRP concentrations. Data are mean ± s.e.m., n = 5, $^{a}p<0.05$; $^{a**}p<0.001$ vs saline; $^{b**}p<0.001$ ipsilateral vs contralateral; $^{b**}p<0.001$ vs CFA. Reproduced with permission from [51].

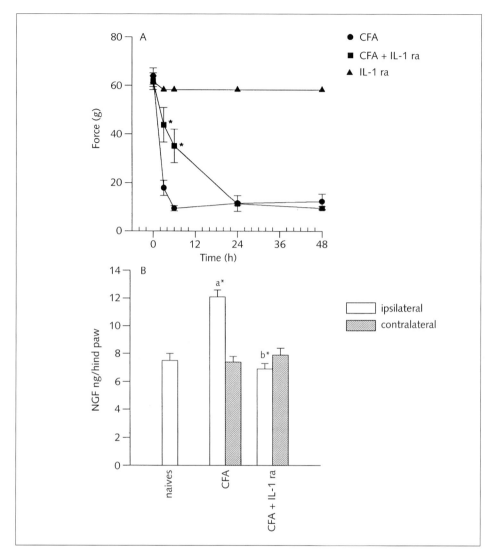

Figure 7
Effect of IL-1ra on CFA-induced mechanical hyperalgesia and concentrations of NGF.
(A) IL-1ra (0.625 μg , i.v, 30 min before and i.p., 6 h after, injection of CFA (100 μl, i.pl.,
squares) reduced the mechanical hyperalgesia measured at 3 h and 6 h after CFA injection
(circles). IL-1ra given alone had no effect on mechanical sensitivity (triangles). The symbols
represent mean ± s.e.m., n = 5, **p<0.01. (B) IL-1ra pretreatment prevented the CFA-
induced increase in NGF concentrations (open columns = ipsilateral; hatched columns = con-
tralateral). Data are mean ± s.e.m., n = 5, [a]*p<0.01 vs naive; [b]*p vs CFA. Reproduced with
permission from [51].

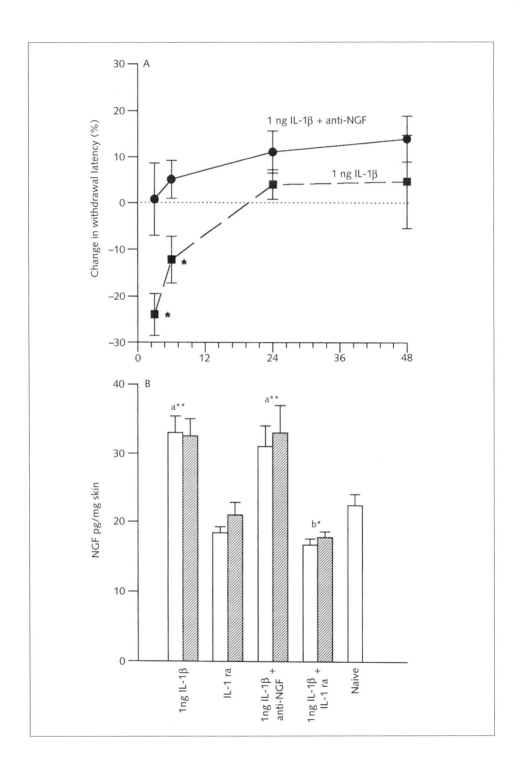

tumour necrosis factor α (TNFα), epidermal growth factor (EGF), and transforming growth factor (TGFα and TGFβ) all increase NGF production by fibroblasts *in vitro* [43, 44]. The increase in NGF during CFA-induced inflammation [7, 24] is important in mediating hyperalgesia because a polyclonal sheep anti-NGF antiserum injected before or after CFA, significantly reduced the increase in sensitivity seen being caused by CFA [7]. Consistent with these observations, a monoclonal anti-NGF antibody brought about similar anti-hypersensitivity effects [51].

Changes in neuropeptide concentrations in CFA-induced inflammatory hyperalgesia

Whether the increase in peptides in the sensory neurons generated during inflammation actually contributes to the behavioural sensory changes is not known. Nociceptive inputs, by virtue of the release of SP and CGRP, have the capacity to increase the excitability of spinal neurons, changing their response characteristics. This phenomenon, called central sensitization, has been shown to play a major role in the generation of post-injury pain hypersensitivity states [38, 74]. NGF, by increasing the concentration of these peptides in the sensory neuron, may increase the capacity of afferents innervating inflamed tissue to produce central sensitization. The changes in peptide expression seen in the DRG during inflammation [7, 24, 35–37] are reflected in an increase in concentrations in the dorsal horn [75, 76] and by an increase in peptide receptor/binding sites in this area [77–79]. Though the fact that doses of dexamethasone and indomethacin that did not prevent hyperalgesia nevertheless suppressed increases in peptide concentrations in the DRG, suggests that the changes in peptide concentration of peptides may not directly reflect changes in acute behavioural sensitivity. A caveat must be that peptide concentrations in the DRG reflect a dynamic interplay between production and transport from the soma. A similar argument could be made about the contribution of IL-1β to inflammatory hypersensitivity. Thus, dexamethasone (smaller dose [51]) substantially reduced

Figure 8
Effect of anti-NGF on IL-1β-induced mechanical hyperalgesia and concentrations of NGF.
*(A) IL-1β (1 ng, i.pl., squares) evoked a significant increase in thermal sensitivity, 3 and 6 h post injection, which was prevented by administration of sheep anti-NGF serum (5 μl g^{-1}, i.p., 1 h before the IL-1β, circles). The asterisks represent significant differences of p<0.01. (B) IL-1β-induced increases in NGF concentrations in the skin both ipsilateral (open columns) and contralateral (hatched columns) to the injection site when measured 48 h later. The increases were prevented by prior administration of IL-1ra (0.625 μg, i.v.). Injection of sheep anti-NGF serum (5 μl g^{-1}, i.p., 1 h before IL-1β) did not affect the increase in NGF concentrations. Data are mean ± s.e.m., n = 4, [a]**p<0.001 vs naive; [b]*p<00.01 vs IL-1β. Reproduced with permission from [51].*

105

(but did not eliminate) the increase in concentrations of IL-1β that followed CFA, but had no effect on behavioural hypersensitivity [51]. In contrast, decreases in inflammatory mechanical hypersensitivity correlated with reductions in concentrations of NGF, achieved using dexamethasone and indomethacin (each at larger doses), or IL-1ra [51]. These findings are consistent with a 'ceiling effect' of IL-1β on the upregulation of NGF and independence in the pathways mediating thermal and mechanical hypersensitivity.

Both dexamethasone and indomethacin reduced neuropeptide concentrations (Fig. 6) at doses below those which affected CFA-induced increases in NGF concentrations (Fig. 4) in the inflamed tissue. This may reflect multiple actions of these anti-inflammatory drugs, including direct effects on the sensory neurons themselves. One possibility is that the drugs interfered with the intracellular signalling action of NGF, once it has bound to *trk* and been transported retrogradely to the soma by, for example, altering the concentrations of transcription factors. There is evidence that dexamethasone can alter neuropeptide concentrations in these neurons. In cultured neonatal rat sensory neurons, for example, corticosterone reduced SP content [80]and, *in vivo*, dexamethasone treatment has been shown to reduce the SP and CGRP content of dental nerves [81], and adrenalectomy resulted in an increase in the SP and CGRP content of rat DRG [82]. The coexistence of neuropeptides and glucocorticoid receptors in the rat spinal and trigeminal ganglia indicates how glucocorticoids could regulate SP and CGRP concentrations without necessarily interfering with the production of target related growth factors/cytokines [83]. Less data is available on non-steroidal anti-inflammatory drug (NSAID) actions on peptide expression in DRG neurons although indomethacin reduces SP concentrations in human ocular aqueous humour [84].

A limited role for eicosanoids in inflammatory hyperalgesia mediated by NGF and IL-1β

The inhibitory effect of glucocorticoids on IL-1β production is fairly well characterized [57, 85–88]. An effect of indomethacin on IL-1β production (by macrophages) was reported only for a very large dose [57]. There are complex interactions among second messenger pathways, steroid hormones, and protooncogenes of the *fos* and *jun* families that converge on the regulation of the NGF gene and several investigators have reported that, in cultured fibroblasts, glucocorticoids inhibited NGF production [80, 89, 90]. Indomethacin acts by inhibiting cyclooxygenase and subsequently PGE_2 synthesis [91]. PGE_2 elicited a dose-dependent increase in NGF mRNA and NGF protein concentrations in rat hippocampal cell cultures [92], but an involvement of eicosanoids in NGF production in peripheral tissues has not been reported. The smaller dose of indomethacin used in the study described above [51] would be expected to have substantially and irreversibly inhibited cyclooxygenase [93] but it had minimal effects on behavioural sensitivity or on concentrations of IL-1β and NGF, suggesting that the effects seen with the larger dose [51] may have been due to some other action of indomethacin.

Both dexamathasone and indomethacin, at doses equivalent to therapeutic doses [93], were surprisingly ineffective in modifying CFA-induced hyperalgesia. Inflammation results in an upregulation of the inducible COX-2 isoform of cyclooxygenase [94], which is readily induced by cytokines including IL-1 [95]. Indomethacin is relatively specific for COX-1 [96] whereas dexamathasone would be expected to prevent the protein synthesis-dependent induction of COX-2 during inflammation [94, 97]. Thus, both the constitutive and the inducible forms of COX should have been inhibited by the indomethacin and dexamethasone but both failed to substantially modify behavioural hypersensitivity, at least compared with neutralisation of NGF [51]. Whether this means that eicosanoids have a limited role in the pathogenesis of CFA-induced sensory hypersensitivity requires further study. That a potent NSAID and a steroid were relatively ineffective in preventing inflammatory hyperalgesia and the upregulation of either IL-1β or NGF may turn out to be related. The only doses of dexamathasone and indomethacin showing anti-hyperalgesic effects were those that prevented an increase in NGF concentrations, supporting a key role for NGF in mediating inflammatory hypersensitivity [51].

The relationship between the upregulation of IL-1β and NGF during inflammation and changes in neuropeptide concentrations and hyperalgesia are complex and a number of apparent inconsistencies between different findings still require explanation, such as the induction of thermal but not mechanical hyperalgesia by IL-1β (given i.pl.) and a reduction of mechanical but not thermal hypersensitivity by IL-1ra administration to CFA-injected animals. This may be the result of complex synergistic interactions between a number of cytokines acting together in concert during inflammation, where one, such as IL-1β, may be necessary but not sufficient in itself to bring about a particular change, a situation quite different from the administration of a single agent in naive animals. Nevertheless, the above data points to a role for IL-1β in the increase in NGF concentration during inflammation and to NGF having an important role in the generation of inflammatory hyperalgesia.

An early role for TNFα in cytokine-NGF interactions

TNFα in the presence and absence of inflammation

TNFα is a 17 kDa cytokine produced by a number of cell types including inflammatory cells (neutrophils, activated lymphocytes, macrophages) and tissue cells (endothelial cells, smooth muscle cells, fibroblasts, basal keratinocytes) [98–101]. This immunomodulating factor has multiple actions including cytolysis, mitogenesis, polymorphonuclear and lymphocyte recruitment as well as initiating a cascade of other cytokines, including IL-1 and IL-6 [101–103]. Concentrations of TNFα increase in disease and immune states including endotoxic shock [104], gout [99], rheumatoid arthritis [102], contact hypersensitivity [105], airway inflammation [103], and immune complex disease [106]. Neutralization of TNFα with antiserum or recombinant TNF receptor-fusion protein molecules reduced the lethality of LPS [107], and attenuated turpentine-induced fever [108] and inflammatory damage in rheumatoid [109] and experimental [110] arthritis. A specific role of TNFα in hyperalgesia has been suggested on the basis of the hypersensitivity produced by local [111] or systemic administration [112] and because of the anti-hyperalgesic action of anti-TNFα antibodies on inflammatory hyperalgesia evoked by bradykinin, LPS and carrageenin [111, 113].

Since TNFα usually precedes IL-1β in the inflammatory cytokine cascade [98], and because this cytokine upregulates NGF *in vitro* [44] and has hyperalgesic actions [111, 112], it was a logical step to investigate whether or not TNFα contributed, via upregulation of IL-1β and NGF, to the establishment of inflammatory hyperalgesia [114].

TNFα, like IL-1β and NGF, was upregulated in the rat hind-paw after the induction of localized peripheral inflammation with CFA. Concentrations of all three mediators were increased by 3 h post CFA injection but the temporal profile of their responses to the inflammation differed. IL-1β concentrations were greatly increased at an early stage (3–6 h) with a gradual decline from their peak over the ensuing five days, NGF concentrations showed an early increase with maintenance at the increased concentration for at least the first five days of the inflammation, and TNFα concentrations increased between 3 and 24 h, at which time they peaked, dipped at 48h and then rose again. The TNFα response was unusual in that TNFα concentrations in contralateral, non-inflamed, hind-paws mirrored (albeit at slightly lower concentrations) those in inflamed (ipsilateral) paws [114]. Although this finding is consistent with a systemic distribution of the cytokine, the failure to detect elevated concentrations of TNFα in the plasma 24 h post CFA injection, when tissue concentrations of the cytokine in both the inflamed (ipsilateral) and non-inflamed (contralateral) paws were at their greatest, argues against systemic distribution [114]. It is possible that the effect in contralateral paws was secondary to systemic spread of some other signal molecule. That detectable basal concentrations of the cytokine were found in the skin in the absence of inflammation was an unexpected finding. Given the reported specificity of the assay used, cross-reactivity with a protein other than TNFα would appear unlikely, although this cannot be excluded. Clearly, this result needs to be confirmed, ideally using ELISA reagents from a different source.

TNFα precedes IL-1β and NGF in inflammatory hyperalgesia induced by CFA

As reported previously [111] TNFα evoked hyperalgesia when injected locally (i.pl.) but the effect, like that of IL-1β [51] or NGF [115], was short-lived and required fairly large doses to elicit changes in sensitivity [114]. These doses did, however, result in local increases in the concentrations of IL-1β and NGF. The increase in concentrations of NGF was likely to have been mediated by the prior upregulation of IL-1β [51], although in culture, TNFα and IL-1β interact synergistically to increase NGF production from non-neuronal cells [44] implying a non-IL-1β dependent action of TNFα on NGF production. TNFα appears, then, to be able to initiate a cytokine cascade, involving IL-1β, that leads to the upregulation of a potent sensitizing agent, NGF.

Pretreatment with anti-NGF antibodies resulted in a marked reduction in CFA-induced hyperalgesia and in the phenotypic changes it produces in primary sensory neurons [7, 116]. Anti-NGF serum also reduced the hyperalgesic effects of both IL-1β [51] and TNFα [114], providing evidence that these two cytokines produce a substantial component of their sensitivity changes via NGF (in the CFA model). Systemic administration of IL-1ra reduced the early phase of CFA-induced hyperalgesia [51]. Anti-TNFα administration also delayed the onset of CFA-induced hyperalgesia with a maximal but incomplete effect on thermal sensitivity at 3 h, and a larger and longer lasting (6 h) effect on mechanical hypersensitivity. By 24 h, however, the hyperalgesia was fully developed in spite of the anti-TNFα treatment. Anti-TNFα administration resulted in a reduction in concentrations of IL-1β but not NGF measured 24 h post-induction of the inflammation (Fig. 9) [114]. It is possible that the short duration of the effects of the sheep anti-TNFα serum on the behavioural hypersensitivity and the failure of the antiserum to affect NGF concentrations at 24 h were the result of injecting too small a dose or of its action being too brief. An alternative explanation is that IL-1β and NGF may be induced during inflammation in TNFα-dependent and TNFα-independent fashions. Consequently, whereas a linear cascade might appear to be operating to produce the transient hyperalgesic effects following the injection of TNFα, the sequence of events is almost certainly more complex, and all the more so in an inflammatory lesion, with multiple events operating over diverse time courses.

Recent evidence indicates that TNFα has a role in inducing the hyperalgesic response to inflammation and this is very likely to be the consequence of its induction of later acting intermediaries, particularly IL-1β and NGF. If TNFα were to be a suitable target for the development of novel analgesics the extent to which IL-1β and NGF upregulation is contingent on prior TNFα upregulation needs to be established. The finding that concentrations of immunoreactive TNFα increased in the non-inflamed hind-paw without any changes in the concentrations of IL-1β and NGF concentrations suggests either that a threshold must exist for TNFα to exert its action in inducing these mediators or that TNFα acts in concert with some other signal molecule(s) which are restricted to the site of the inflammation.

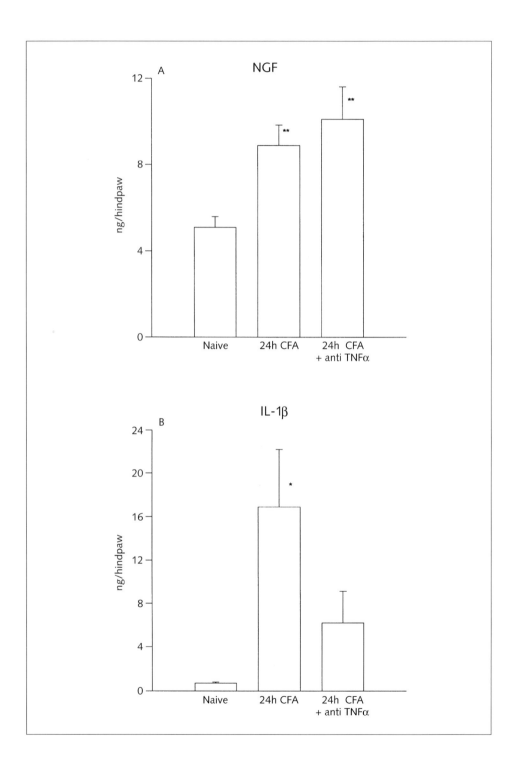

Leukaemia inhibitory factor (LIF) as an anti-inflammatory and anti-hyperalgesic cytokine

Interactions of LIF with inflammatory mediators

Leukemia inhibitory factor is a neuropoietic cytokine involved in both the neural and immune responses to injury and concentrations of LIF are increased in a variety of inflammatory conditions [117–123]. Administration of LIF can suppress inflammatory signs in certain situations [120], for instance in intratracheal LPS-induced inflammation [122]. Also, LIF increased corticosterone concentrations via an effect upon the hypothalamo-pituitary adrenal axis [124]. However, other evidence suggests that LIF can also act as a pro-inflammatory cytokine. Exogenously added LIF induced expression of acute-phase proteins [125, 126] and stimulated the production of pro-inflammatory cytokines and monocyte chemoattactants [121, 127, 128]. Passive immunoneutralization of LIF protected mice against the lethal effects of endotoxin and inhibited LPS-induced increases in circulating IL-1 and IL-6 [129], and injection of large doses of LIF into skin or joints produced swelling and leukocyte invasion [130, 131].

In the nervous system, concentrations of LIF mRNA increased markedly soon after injury [132–134], and experiments with LIF null mutant mice revealed that LIF was required for some of the striking changes in neuronal gene expression that are characteristic of the response to injury [135–137]. Lack of LIF led to premature neuronal death [138] and a diminished rate of immune cell influx following peripheral nerve injury [139]. LIF and its receptors (LIF-R and gp130) are abundantly expressed in pituitary cells and LIF acts in a paracrine fashion to regulate release of adrenocorticotrophin and growth hormone release [138–140]. Consequently, while LIF appears to be an important modulator of inflammatory events and their interaction with the nervous system, there is contradictory evidence as to whether the overall net effect of this cytokine is pro-or anti-inflammatory.

LIF limits NGF-mediated inflammatory hyperalgesia

A recent study [141] provided good evidence that LIF is produced during CFA-induced cutaneous inflammation and acts to limit the inflammation and inflamma-

Figure 9
Effect of anti-TNFα on CFA-induced increases in concentrations of NGF and IL-1β.
The effect of a single injection of sheep anti-TNFα serum (5 μl kg⁻¹, 1 h before CFA) on increases in concentrations of (a) NGF and (b) IL-1β, measured in hind-paws, 24 h after injection of CFA (100 μl, i.pl.). The anti TNF(serum failed to prevent the increase in NGF concentrations but diminished increases in concentrations of IL-1β. Values shown are mean ± s.e.m., n = 4, **p < 0.01 naive vs treated. Reproduced with permission from [114].

tory hyperalgesia. The absence of LIF exacerbated the inflammatory response to CFA, whereas increased concentrations of LIF, brought about by its injection, abrogated a number of the effects of the CFA [141]. Inflammatory oedema has both neurogenic and non-neurogenic components. The former are due to an efferent function of sensory neurons releasing vasoactive neuropeptides as part of the axon-reflex [142, 143], whereas the latter are the consequence of the direct action of inflammatory mediators on the vasculature and capillary permeability. While it is not clear which component was responsible for the exaggerated response of LIF knockout to CFA [141], the failure of exogenous LIF to reduce swelling, while diminishing concentrations of IL-1β and NGF, indicates an early divergence of the inflammatory pathways involved. A large dose of LIF (1 mg) caused swelling in the goat radiocarpal joint [130] and injection of LIF (at >100 ng) directly into the ear pinna of mice increased ear thickness, although by a much smaller extent than a 250-fold lower dose of IL-1α [131]. Further, injection of a large dose of LIF (1 mg) into non-inflamed juvenile rats (12 days old) caused a prolonged hypersensitivity to mechanical stimulation[144]. In contrast, small doses of LIF (up to 100 ng), injected into non-inflamed hind-paws in adult rats did not evoke mechanical hypersensitivity [141]. Either the difference in dose or in the age of the animals may account for the different results. It is also possible that small doses of LIF are anti-inflammatory whereas larger doses, perhaps acting via the receptors for other members of the cytokine family with which LIF shares the gp130 signal-transducing subunit [145] are pro-inflammatory. Whatever explanation applies, caution is needed in interpreting the pro-inflammatory effects of large doses of exogenous LIF, which may have pharmacological actions different from those of endogenous LIF. The need for such caution is emphasised by the results obtained with the LIF knockout animals [141].

LIF suppressed CFA-induced up-regulation of both IL-1β and NGF and deletion of LIF led to an amplified induction of these proteins, suggesting a role for LIF in regulating the cytokine cascade at an early stage in the inflammatory process [141]. LIF appears to have the opposite effect in chondrocytes, where it increased concentrations of IL-1, IL-6 and IL-8 [127]. Although the cellular target for LIF action in skin remains to be identified, LIF presumably exerts its anti-inflammatory effect via the Jak-STAT pathway [145]. This could lead to inhibition of the transcription or release of a pro-inflammatory cytokine such as IL-1 or to the release of an endogenous anti-inflammatory agent such as IL-1ra [146]. Regarding likely inducers of LIF, TNFα induced LIF in dermal cultures [147].

In summary, the mRNA for LIF was elevated during skin inflammation produced by CFA (injected i.pl.). Further, while LIF knockout mice displayed normal sensitivity to cutaneous mechanical and thermal stimulation compared with wild-type mice, the degree of CFA-induced inflammation in mice lacking LIF was increased in spatial extent, amplitude, cellular infiltrate and in expression of IL-1β and NGF. Conversely, local injection of LIF diminished CFA-induced mechanical and thermal hypersensitivity and production of IL-1β and NGF. These data show that up-regulation of LIF during peripheral inflammation serves a key, early anti-inflammatory role and that exogenous LIF is anti-hyperalgesic [141]. While gp130 and LIF receptor agonists might be considered as novel anti-inflammatory and anti-hyperalgesic targets, stimulation (or antagonism) of gp130 should not to be taken lightly, in view of the other important ligands that utilize it as a transducing element [145].

Peripheral cell types contributing to IL-1β-NGF interactions

The role of NGF in the various components of inflammatory hyperalgesia
Inflammatory pain is a multifaceted syndrome that comprises three distinct components: spontaneous pain referred to the site of the inflammation, an amplification of the response to noxious stimuli, hyperalgesia, and finally the generation of pain by what would normally be innocuous stimuli, allodynia. These last two components manifest both in the inflamed tissue (primary zone) and in the surrounding non-inflamed tissue (secondary zone). A number of different mechanisms, operating at different times and at different locations, contribute to inflammatory pain. Direct activation of chemosensitive nociceptors by irritants or inflammatory mediators elicits spontaneous pain [148], an alteration in the transduction sensitivity of nociceptors by sensitizing mediators like bradykinin and PGE_2 contributes to primary hyperalgesia [149] whereas sensory input to the spinal cord, as a result of the release of excitatory amino acids and neuropeptides, sensitizes central neurones in an NMDA-receptor and tachykinin receptor mediated fashion, to produce secondary hyperalgesia and allodynia [150, 151].

It is now recognised that neurological dysfunction in the mature nervous system can occur not only as a result of neurotrophin deficiency, but also as a result of excess. NGF may contribute to inflammatory hypersensitivity by producing both local and central changes in sensitivity.

Mast cell degranulation, NGF, IL-1β and inflammatory hyperalgesia
NGF produced in peripheral tissue [64] acts on those cells in the tissue which express the high affinity protein tyrosine kinase NGF receptor *trkA* [152, 153]. TrkA is present on inflammatory cells as well as on sympathetic cells and a sub-population of small-diameter sensory neurons [154–157]. A cytokine-like action of NGF on inflammatory cells was described some years ago [158] and includes effects on mast cells, basophils, lymphocytes and neutrophils leading to proliferation and cytokine production [13, 27–31, 159, 160]. While these actions may act to amplify the inflammatory response they may also contribute indirectly to sensitivity changes by causing the release of inflammatory mediators which then act directly on sensory nerve terminals. Mast cells, which have a major role in immediate-type hypersensitivity reactions and contribute to chronic inflammation [162], are particularly

important targets for NGF. NGF promotes their survival [163], growth [31], differentiation [160] and degranulation [32, 33, 164].

Acute degranulation of mast cells releases a number of proteinases, cytokines and amines, including 5-hydroxytryptamine and histamine [165], each of which could sensitize nociceptors, either directly or indirectly via the breakdown of precursor proteins or by inducing the release of inflammatory mediators from other cell types. Chronic degranulation of mast cells with compound 48/80 [166], by depleting the cells of amines and other inflammatory mediators, might be interfering with the normal sensitizing consequences of an NGF action on mast cells and in this way attenuate inflammatory hyperalgesia. However, this may not necessarily mean that the role of the mast cell in inflammation relates only to an action of NGF on these cells. Mast cells are also a potential source of NGF production [25] and recently it was shown that chronic degranulation of mast cells inhibited an increase in NGF during inflammation above the concentrations in non-inflamed animals treated with compound 48/80 [115]. This may reflect an impairment in the synthesis, storage or release of NGF from mast cells or a reduction in the release of a cytokine, such as TNFα, from the mast cells, which acts on other cell types to produce NGF [44]. The concentrations of IL-1β, which is a powerful inducer of NGF [51, 65], were not affected by 48/80 treatment [115]. The failure to increase NGF concentrations during inflammation may contribute to the maintained reduction of inflammatory hyperalgesia in these animals. This finding contrasts with the transient effects of compound 48/80 treatment on the hyperalgesia produced by systemic NGF, which appear to be due entirely to a reduction in amine release [8].

Sympathectomy, NGF, IL-1β and inflammatory hyperalgesia

Sympathetic neurons are prototypic examples of NGF-responsive neurons [167] and their survival is dependent on access to NGF during development [157]. Removal of postganglionic sympathetic terminals by chemical sympathectomy with guanethidine resulted in an increase in the basal concentrations of NGF in the skin (Fig. 10) [115]. This result suggests either that these cells utilize a considerable component of the normal constitutive production of NGF or that some element of sympathetic innervation of the periphery suppresses NGF production by target tissue. The ele-

Figure 10
Effect of sympathectomy on concentrations of IL-1β and NGF.
Sympathectomy did not alter the inflammatory upregulation of IL-1β and NGF measured 48 h after CFA injections, but did result in an increase in basal concentrations of NGF [°°,°°° ipsilateral vs contralateral p < 0.01, < 0.001,**, *** , ipsilateral (CFA) vs naive or ipsilateral (CFA + sympath.) vs sympathectomized non-inflamed (Sympath.) p < 0.01, < 0.001)]. Reproduced with permission from [115].

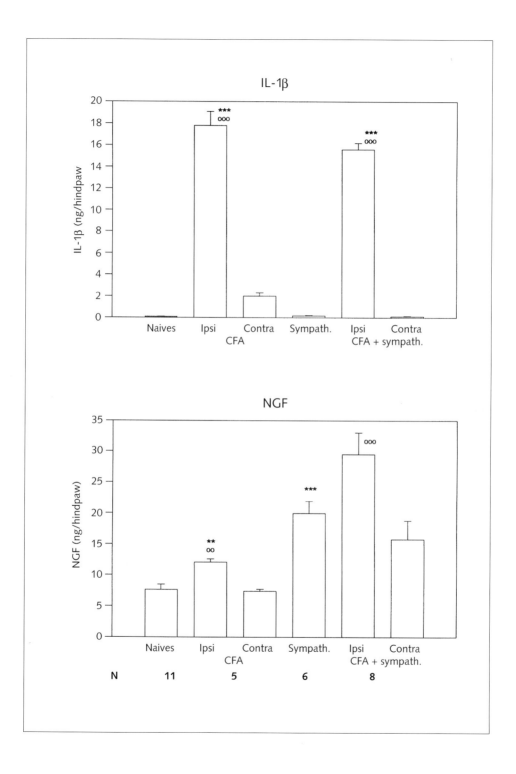

vation in basal NGF may have contributed to the increased thermal sensitivity measured in sympathectomized animals (Figs. 11 and 12) [115], a finding that is consistent with the increased thermal sensitivity in transgenic mice engineered to overexpress NGF in the skin using a keratin promoter [168]. The increase in basal (i.e. unstimulated) concentrations of NGF in sympathectomized animals resulted only in a thermal hyperalgesia whereas in inflammation there is both mechanical and thermal hyperalgesia. This may partly reflect the dose of NGF used. Small doses of NGF (2–20 ng, given i.pl.) evoked thermal but not mechanical hyperalgesia whereas larger doses (200 ng) evoked both [7]. Another possibility is that NGF alone dose not mediate all the changes in sensitivity that occur during inflammation. A dissociation between thermal and mechanical hyperalgesia evoked by NGF has been observed previously [8].

The absence of an increase in basal IL-1β concentrations in sympathectomized rats indicates that the increases in basal NGF concentrations were not caused by increased concentrations of this cytokine [115]. NGF upregulation above basal concentrations during inflammation was not affected by sympathectomy (Fig. 10) [115], and sympathectomy reduced only the earliest phase of inflammatory hypersensitivity, with the hyperalgesia present at 6 to 48 h after CFA treatment left unaffected (Fig. 11) [115]. This may appear surprising in view of the sympathetic-dependence of the hyperalgesia evoked by NGF given i.pl. [115, 169]. The reason for this is likely to be related to timing. Local NGF administration elevated NGF concentration in the target for only a very brief period and produced a short-lasting hyperalgesia, whereas in CFA-induced inflammation NGF concentrations are increased for at least several days and the hyperalgesia was persistent. Different mechanisms may operate at different times. NGF may have a *trkA*-mediated action on sympathetic terminals in the periphery, which leads to a shortlasting hyperalgesia whenever NGF concentrations rise acutely. Sympathetic terminals can produce hyperalgesia by releasing eicosanoids or other mediators which sensitize sensory neurons [170]. A sympathetic-dependent hyperalgesia manifests for several hours after local NGF administration (Fig. 12) [115] and during the earliest phase of CFA-induced inflammation (Fig. 11) [115]. Subsequently, a non sympathetic-dependent component contributes to inflammatory hyperalgesia, although this component is NGF-dependent. The time-dependent nature of the involvement of the sympathetic nervous system in inflammatory hyperalgesia may explain the different results in favour of [111, 170, 171] and against [172–174] a sympathetic-dependence of inflammatory hyperalgesia, although the mechanism of the NGF-dependent contribution to the sympathetic-independent component of inflammatory hyperalgesia remains to be elucidated.

A role for NGF in the early and later phases of inflammatory hyperalgesia
Both sympathectomy and mast cell degranulation had maximal efficacy in reducing inflammatory hyperalgesia in the first few hours after the onset of inflammation

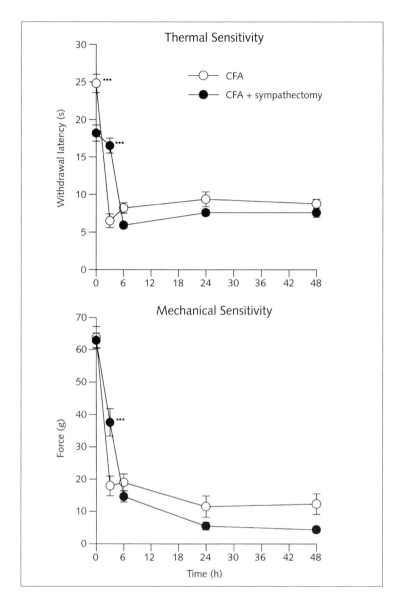

Figure 11
Effect of sympathectomy on CFA-induced thermal and mechanical hyperalgesia.
Effect of sympathectomy (filled circles) on CFA-induced (100 μl, i.pl., open circles) thermal
and mechanical hyperalgesia, assessed by 50° C hotplate response latency and the flexion
withdrawal reflex mechanical threshold, respectively; n = 5 for CFA group; n = 9 for sympa-
*thectomized animals, ***p < 0.001 CFA vs CFA + sympathectomy groups). Reproduced with*
permission from [115].

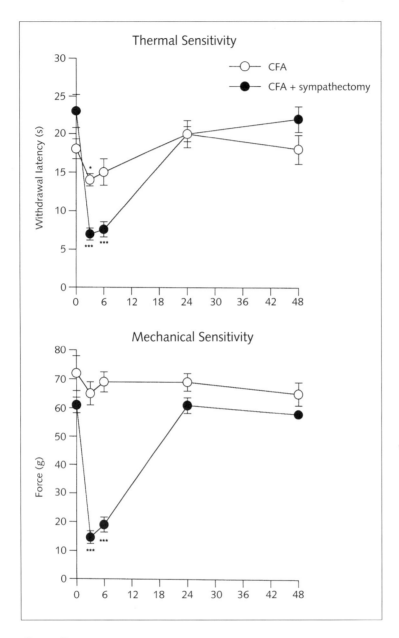

Figure 12
Effect of sympathectomy on NGF-induced thermal and mechanical hyperalgesia.
Sympathectomy (open circles) reduced the transient sensitivity increase evoked by NGF
*(200 ng, i.pl., filled circles), *,***p < 0.05, < 0.001, n = 5 for CFA group; n = 4 for CFA + sym-*
pathectomy. Reproduced with permission from [115].

[115]. This is a time when any change must necessarily be restricted to the site of the inflammation since the retrograde transport of NGF in sensory neurons from the hind-paw to the L4 and L5 dorsal root ganglia takes 5–7 h [48], even before any transcriptional change is effected. While peripheral sensitization may continue to contribute beyond this time, changes at the dorsal root ganglia are likely also to be important. NGF, once it reaches the cell bodies of *trkA* expressing sensory neurons in the dorsal root ganglia, will, by activating specific signal transduction pathways [175], cause alterations in phenotype. This includes the upregulation of neuropeptides, growth factors and Na$^+$ channels [16, 24, 42, 176]. All of these could contribute to inflammatory hypersensitivity in a number of ways. By promoting peripheral sprouting and the hyperinnervation of inflamed tissue [42], augmenting neurogenic inflammation following the upregulation of SP [177] and, finally, increasing the central synaptic action of sensory neurons as a result of an increase or novel release of neuropeptide neuromodulators from the central terminals of afferents in the dorsal horn of the spinal cord. Inflammation results in a substantial increase in the numbers of DRG neurons expressing preprotachykinin A and CGRP mRNA and in the concentrations of the peptides (SP and CGRP) in the sensory neurons [36, 45, 51], and these changes are NGF-dependent [7, 24, 42]. An increase in the concentrations of the neuropeptides may augment the central sensitization normally produced by C-afferent inputs into the spinal cord [178, 179] and in this way contribute to inflammatory hypersensitivity.

In summary, in the early phase of inflammation the contribution of NGF to inflammatory hypersensitivity is due exclusively to a peripheral action which is markedly attenuated by either depletion of mast cell granules or sympathectomy. The subsequent phases of inflammatory hypersensitivity are independent of the sympathetic nervous system but remain NGF-dependent and are likely to reflect both a peripheral action and transcription-dependent changes in the function of sensory neurons. [115].

Conclusions

Further research into the interactions between inflammation and the nervous system (see Fig. 13) must help in the understanding of the changes that the former produces in the latter and, hopefully, such work will lead to the development of more effective drugs to prevent or inhibit inflammatory hyperalgesia and abnormal pain sensitivity. Certainly drugs which interfere with the production or action of NGF may offer a new class of inflammation-specific analgesics. Also, unravelling the cytokine response to inflammation may offer novel therapeutic options, e.g. LIF-mimics and inhibitors of TNFα and IL-1β, for managing local inflammation. However, the quest for such agents will not be straightforward because polypeptides/proteins such as NGF, TNFα, IL-1β and LIF are not small molecules

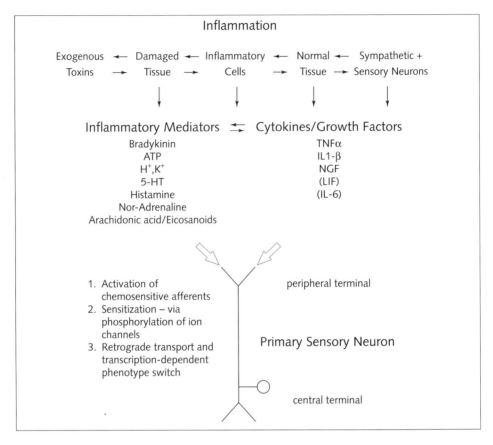

Figure 13
The postulated roles of cytokines, other hyperalgesic agents and inhibitors of these media-
tors in inflammation. TNFα = tumour necrosis factor α, IL-1β = interleukin-1β, NGF = nerve
growth factor, LIF = leukaemia inhibitory factor, IL-6 = interleukin-6.

that readily yield up the characteristics of their interactions with their receptors, and some of those receptors share signalling elements with other important cytokines and hormones.

Acknowledgements
We thank the MRC, the EU (BMH4-CT95-0172) and the Human Frontier Science Program for financial support.

References

1   Woolf CJ (1996) Phenotypic modification of primary sensory neurones: the role of nerve growth factor in the production of persistent pain. *Phil Trans Roy Soc Lond* B, 351: 441–448

2   Hokfelt T, Zhang X, Wiesenfeld-Hallin Z (1994) Messenger plasticity in primary sensory neurons following axotomy and its functional implications. *TINS* 17(1): 22–30

3   Verge VMK, Richardson PM, Wiesenfeld-Hallin Z, Hokfelt T (1995) Differential influence of nerve growth factor on neuropeptide expression *in vivo*: a novel role in peptide suppression in adult sensory neurons. *J Neurosci* 15: 2081–2096

4   Reeh PW (1994) Chemical excitation and sensitization of nociceptors. In: L Urban (ed): *Cellular mechanisms of sensory processing. NATO ASI series.* Cell Biology Vol 79. Springer-Verlag, Berlin, Heidelberg, 119–131

5   Treede R-D, Meyer RA, Raja SN, Campbell JN (1992) Peripheral and central mechanisms of cutaneous hyperalgesia. *Prog Neurobiol* 38: 397–421

6   Gold MS, Reichling DB, Schuster MJ, Levine JD (1996) Hyperalgesic agents increase a tetrodotoxin-resistant Na^+ current in nociceptors. *Proc Natl Acad Sci USA* 93: 1108–1112

7   Woolf CJ, Safieh-Garabedian B, Ma Q-P, Crilly P, Winter J (1994) Nerve growth factor contributes to the generation of inflammatory sensory hypersensitivity. *Neurosci* 62: 327–331

8   Lewin GR, Rueff A, Mendell LM (1994) Peripheral and central mechanisms of NGF-induced hyperalgesia. *Eur J Neurosci* 6: 1903–1912

9   Johnson EM, Jr, Rich KM, Yip HK (1986) The role of NGF in sensory neurons *in vivo*. *TINS* 9: 33–37

10   Barde Y-A (1989) Trophic factors and neuronal survival. *Neuron* 2: 1525–1534

11   Korsching S (1993) The neurotrophic factor concept: A reexamination. *J Neurosci* 13: 2739–2748

12   Rich KM, Luszczynski JR, Osbourne PA, Johnson EM, Jr (1987) Nerve growth factor protects adult sensory neurons from cell death and atrophy caused by nerve injury. *J Neurocytol* 16: 261–268

13   Matsuda H, Coughlin MD, Bienenstock J, Denburg JA (1988) Nerve growth factor promotes human hemopoietic colony growth and differentiation. *Proc Natl Acad Sci USA* 85: 6508–6512

14   Chao MV (1992) Neurotrophin receptors: a window into neuronal differentiation. *Neuron* 9: 583–593

15   Glass DJ, Yancopoulos GD (1993) The neurotrophins and their receptors. *Trends Cell Biol* 3: 262–268

16   Lindsay RM, Harmar AJ (1989) Nerve growth factor regulates expression of neuropeptide genes in adult sensory neurons. *Nature* 337: 362–364

17   Gold BG, Mobley WC, Matheson SF (1991) Regulation of axonal caliber, neurofilament

content and nuclear localization in mature sensory neurons by nerve growth factor. *J Neurosci* 11: 943–955

18   Lindsay RM, Lockett C, Sternberg J, Winter J (1989) Neuropeptide expression in cultures of adult sensory neurons: modulation of substance P and calcitonin gene-related peptide levels by nerve growth factor. *Neurosci* 33: 53–65

19   Rich KM, Yip HK, Osbourne PA, Schmidt RF, Johnson EM, Jr (1984) Role of nerve growth factor in the adult dorsal root ganglia neuron and its response to injury. *J Comp Neurol* 230: 110–118

20   Lewin GR, Mendell LM (1993) Nerve growth factor and nociception. *TINS* 16: 353

21   Lewin GR, Ritter AM, Mendell LM (1993) Nerve growth factor-induced hyperalgesia in the neonatal and adult rat. *J Neurosci* 13(5): 2136–2148

22   Weskamp G, Otten U (1987) An enzyme-linked immunoassay for nerve growth factor (NGF): a tool for studying regulatory mechanisms involved in NGF production in brain and in peripheral tissues. *J Neurochem* 48: 1779–1786

23   Varilek GW, Weinstock JV, Pantazis NJ (1992) Isolated hepatic granulomas from mice infected with Schistosome mansoni contain nerve growth factor. *Infection Immunity* 59: 4443–4449

24   Donnerer J, Schuligoi R, Stein C (1992) Increased content and transport of substance P and calcitonin gene-related peptide in sensory nerves innervating inflamed tissue: evidence for a regulatory function of nerve growth factor *in vivo*. *Neurosci* 49(3): 693–698

25   Leon A, Buriani A, Dal Toso R, Fabris M, Romanello S, Aloe L, Levi-Montalcini R (1994) Mast cells synthesize, store, and release nerve growth factor. *Proc Natl Acad Sci USA* 91: 3739–3743

26   Thorpe LW, Stach RW, Morgan B, Perez-Polo JR (1988) The influence of nerve growth factor on the *in vitro* proliferative response of rat spleen lymphocytes. *J Neurosci* Res 18: 134

27   Otten U, Ehrhard P, Peck R (1987) Nerve growth factor induces growth and differentiation of human B lymphocytes. *Proc Natl Acad Sci USA* 86: 10059–10063

28   Bischoff SC, Dahinden CA (1992) Effect of nerve growth factor on the release of inflammatory mediators by mature human basophils. *Blood* 79: 2662–2669

29   Horigome K, Pryor JC, Bullock ED, Johnson EM, Jr (1993) Mediator release from mast cells by nerve growth factor. Neurotrophin specificity and receptor mediation. *J Biol Chem* 268: 14881–14887

30   Bohm A, Aloe L, Levi-Montalcini R (1986) Nerve growth factor enhances precocious differentiation and numerical increase in mast cells in cultures of rat splenocytes. *Accad Naz Lincei* 80: 1

31   Aloe L, Levi-Montalcini R (1977) Mast cell increase in tissue of neonatal rats injected with nerve growth factor. *Brain Res* 133: 358–366

32   Mazurek N, Weskamp G, Erne P, Otten U (1986) Nerve growth factor induces mast cell degranulation without changing intracellular calcium levels. *FEBS Lett* 198: 315–320

33   Pearce FL, Thompson HL (1986) Some characteristics of histamine secretion from rat peritoneal mast cells stimulated with nerve growth factor. *J Physiol Lond* 372: 379–393

34   Lee Y, Takami K, Kawal Y, Girgis S, Hillyard CJ, Macintyre I, Emson PC, Tohyama M (1985) Distribution of calcitonin gene-related peptide in the rat peripheral nervous system with reference to its coexistence with substance P. *Neurosci* 15: 1227–1237

35   Noguchi K, Morita Y, Kiyama H, Ono K, Tohyama M (1988) A noxious stimulus induces the preprotachykinin-A gene expression in the rat dorsal root ganglion: a quantitative study using in situ hybridization histochemistry. *Mol Brain Res* 4: 31–35

36   Donaldson LF, Harmar AJ, McQueen DS, Seckl JR (1992) Increased expression of preprotachykinin, calcitonin gene-related peptide, but not vasoactive intestinal polypeptide messenger RNA in dorsal root ganglia during the development of adjuvant monoarthritis in the rat. *Mol Brain Res* 16: 143–149

37   Smith GD, Harmar AJ, McQueen DS, Seckl JR (1992) Increase in substance P and CGRP, but not somatostatin content of innervating dorsal root ganglia in adjuvant monoarthritis in the rat. *Neurosci Lett* 137: 257–260

38   Woolf CJ (1991) Generation of acute pain: central mechanisms. *Brit Med Bull* 47: 523–533

39   Sivilotti LG, Woolf CJ (1994) The contribution of GABAA and glycine receptors to central sensitization: disinhibition and touch-evoked allodynia in the spinal cord. *J Neurophysiol* 72 169–179

40   Della Seta D, de Acetis L, Aloe L, Alleva E (1994) NGF effects on hot plate behaviors in mice. *Pharmacol Biochem Behav* 49: 701–705

41   Petty BG, Cornblath DR, Adornato BT, Chaudhry V, Flexner C, Wachsman M, Sinicropi D, Burton LE, Peroutka SJ (1994) The effect of systemically administered recombinant human nerve growth factor in healthy human subjects. *Ann Neurol* 36: 244–246

42   Leslie TA, Emson PC, Dowd PM, Woolf CJ (1995) Nerve growth factor contributes to the upregulation of GAP-43 and preprotachykinin A mRNA in primary sensory neurons following peripheral inflammation. *Neurosci* 67: 753–761

43   Matsuoka I, Meyer M, Thoenen H (1991) Cell type specify regulation of nerve growth factor (NGF) synthesis in nonneuronal cells – comparison of Schwann cells with other cell types. *J Neurosci* 11: 3165–3177

44   Hattori A, Tanaka E, Murase K, Ishida N, Chatani Y, Tsujimoto M, Hayashi K, Kohno M (1993) Tumor necrosis factor stimulates the synthesis and secretion of biologically active nerve growth factor in non-neuronal cells. *J Biol Chem* 268: 2577–2582

45   Heumann R, Korsching S, Bandtlow C, Thoenen H (1987) Changes of nerve growth factor synthesis in nonneuronal cells in response to sciatic nerve transection. *J Cell Biol* 104: 1623–1631

46   Aloe L, Tuveri MA, Levi-Montalcini R (1992) Studies on carrageenan-induced arthritis in adult rats: presence of nerve growth factor and role of sympathetic innervation. *Rheumatol Int* 12: 213–216

47   Constantinou J, Reynolds ML, Woolf CJ, Safieh-Garabedian B, Fitzgerald M (1994) Nerve growth factor levels in developing rat skin; upregulation following skin wounding. *Neurorep* 5(17): 2281–2284

48   DiStefano PS, Friedman B, Radziejewesk C, Alexander C, Boland P, Schieck CM, Lind-

say RM, Wiegand SJ (1992) The neurotrophins BDNF, NT-3 and NGF display distinct patterns of retrograde axonal transport in peripheral and central neurons. *Neuron* 8: 983–993

49   McMahon SB, Armanini MP, Ling LH, Phillips HS (1994) Expression and coexpression of *trk* receptors in subpopulations of adult primary sensory neurons projecting to identified peripheral targets. *Neuron* 12: 1161–1171

50   McMahon SB, Bennett DLH, Priestley JV, Shelton DL (1995) The biological effects of endogenous NGF in adult sensory neurones revealed by a *trkA* IgG fusion molecule. *Nature Med* 1: 774–780

51   Safieh-Garabedian B, Poole S, Allchorne A, Winter J, Woolf CJ (1995) Contribution of interleukin-1β to the inflammation-induced increase in nerve growth factor levels and inflammatory hyperalgesia. *Br J Pharmacol* 115: 1265–1275

52   Movat HZ (1987) Tumor necrosis factor and interleukin-1; their role in acute inflammation and microvascular injury. *J Lab Clin Med* 110: 668–681

53   Dinarello CA (1991) Interleukin-1 and interleukin-1 antagonism. *Blood* 8: 1627–1652

54   Bianchi M, Sacerdote P, Locatelli L, Mantegazza P, Panerai AE (1992) Corticotrophin releasing hormone, interleukin-1-alpha and tumor necrosis factor-alpha share characteristics of stress mediators. *Brain Res* 546: 139–142

55   Libby P, Ordovas JM, Auger KR, Robbins AH, Birinyi LK, Dinarello CA (1986) Endotoxin and tumour necrosis factor induce interleukin-1 gene expression in human vascular endothelial cells. *Am J Pathol* 124: 179–185

56   Arai K, Lee F, Miyajima A, Miyataki S, Arai N, Yokota T (1990) Cytokines: Coordinators of immune and inflammatory responses. *Ann Rev Biochem* 59: 783–836

57   Dawson J, Rordorf-Adam C, Geiger T, Towbin H, Kunz S, Nguyen H, Zingel O (1993) Interleukin-1 (IL-1) production in a mouse tissue chamber model of inflammation. II. Identification of (tissue) macrophages as the IL-1 producing cells and the effect of anti-inflammatory drugs. *Agents Actions* 38: 255–264

58   Ferreira SH, Lorenzetti BB, Bristow AF, Poole S (1988) Interleukin-1 beta as a potent hyperalgesic agent antagonized by a tripeptide analogue. *Nature* 334: 698–700

59   Schweizer A, Feige U, Fontana A, Muller K, Dinarello CA (1988) Interleukin-1 enhances pain reflexes. Mediation through increased prostaglandin E2 levels. *Agents Actions* 25: 246–251

60   Ferreira SH (1993) The role of interleukins and nitric oxide in the mediation of inflammatory pain and its control by peripheral analgesics. *Drugs* 46 (Suppl 1): 1–9

61   Fukuoka H, Kawatani M, Hisamitsu R, Takeshige C (1994) Cutaneous hyperalgesia induced by peripheral injection of interleukin-1β in the rat. *Brain Res* 657: 133–140

62   Watkins LR, Wiertelak EP, Goehler L, Smith KP, Martin D, Maier SF (1994) Characterization of cytokine-induced hyperalgesia. *Brain Res*, 654: 15–26

63   Perkins MN, Kelly D, Davis AJ (1995) Bradykinin B1 and B2 receptor mechanisms and cytokine-induced hyperalgesia in the rat. *Can J Physiol Pharmacol* 73: 832–836

64   Bandtlow C, Heumann R, Schwab ME, Thoenen H (1987) Cellular localization of nerve growth factor synthesis by in situ hybridization. *EMBO J* 6: 891–899

65   Lindholm D, Neumann R, Meyer M, Thoenen H (1987) Interleukin-1 regulates synthesis of nerve growth factor in non-neuronal cells of rat sciatic nerve. *Nature* 330: 658–659

66   Lindholm D, Heumann R, Hengerer B, Thoenen H (1988) Interleukin-1 increases stability and transcription of mRNA encoding nerve growth factor in cultured rat fibroblasts. *J Biol Chem* 263: 16348–16351

67   Yoshida K, Gage FH (1992) Cooperative regulation of nerve growth factor synthesis and secretion in fibroblasts and astrocytes by fibroblast growth factor and other cytokines. *Brain Res* 569: 14–25

68   McQuay HJ, Carroll D, Moore RA (1988) Post-operative orthopaedic pain – the effect of opiate premedication and local anesthetic blocks. *Pain* 33: 291–295

69   Crestani F, Seguy F, Dantzer R (1991) Behavioural effects of peripherally injected interleukin-1: role of prostaglandins. *Brain Res* 542: 330–335

70   Follenfant RL, Nakamura-Craig M, Henderson B, Higgs GA (1989) Inhibition by neuropeptides of interleukin-1β-induced, prostaglandin-independent hyperalgesia. *Br J Pharmacol* 98: 41–43

71   Davis AJ, Perkins MN (1994) The involvement of bradykinin B1 and B2 receptor mechanisms in cytokine-induced mechanical hyperalgesia in the rat. *Br J Pharmacol* 113: 63–68

72   Hart RP, Shadiack AM, Jonakait GM (1991) Substance P gene expression is regulated by interleukin-1 in cultured sympathetic ganglia. *J Neurosci Res* 29: 282–291

73   Shadiack AM, Hart RP, Carlson CD, Jonakait GM (1993) Interleukin-1 induces substance P in sympathetic ganglia through the induction of leukemia inhibitory factor (LIF). *J Neurosci* 13(6): 2601–2609

74   Woolf CJ (1983) Evidence for a central component of post-injury pain hypersensitivity. *Nature* 306: 686–688

75   Oku R, Satoh M, Takagi H (1987) Release of substance P from the spinal dorsal horn is enhanced in polyarthritic rats. *Neurosci Lett* 74: 315–319

76   Schaible H-G, Jarrott B, Hope PJ, Duggan AW (1990) Release of immunoreactive substance P in the spinal cord during development of acute arthritis in the knee joint of the cat: a study with antibody microprobes. *Brain Res* 529: 214–223

77   Kar S, Rees RG, Quirion R (1993) Altered calcitonin gene-related peptide, substance P and enkephalin immunoreactivities and receptor binding sites in the dorsal spinal cord of the polyarthritic rat. *Eur J Neurosci* 6: 345–354

78   Schafer MK-H, Nohr D, Krause JE, Weihe E (1993) Inflammation-induced upregulation of NK1 receptor mRNA in dorsal horn neurones. *Neurorep* 4: 1007–1010

79   Stucky CL, Galeazza MT, Seybold VS (1993) Time-dependent changes in Bolton-Hunter labelled 125I-substance P binding in rat spinal cord following unilateral adjuvant-induced peripheral inflammation. *Neurosci* 57: 397–409

80   Maclean DB, Bennett B, Morris M, Wheeler FB (1989) Differential regulation of calcitonin gene-related peptide and substance P in cultured neonatal rat vagal sensory neurones. *Brain Res* 478: 349–355

81   Hong D, Byers MR, Oswald RJ (1993) Dexamethasone treatment reduces sensory neu-ropeptides and nerve sprouting reactions in injured teeth. *Pain* 55: 171–181

82   Smith GD, Seckl JR, Sheward WJ, Bennie JG, Caroll SM, Dick H, Harmar AJ (1991) Effect of adrenalectomy and dexamethasone on neuropeptide content of dorsal root ganglia in the rat. *Brain Res* 564: 27–30

83   Deleon M, Covenas R, Chadi G, Narvaez JA, Fuxe K, Cintra A (1994) Subpopulations of primary sensory neurones show coexistence of neuropeptides and glucocorticoid receptors in the rat spinal and trigeminal ganglia. *Brain Res* 636: 338–342

84   Kieselbach G, Troger J, Kaehler C, Saria A (1993) Indomethacin reduces substance P levels in human ocular aqueous humor. *Eur J Pharmacol* 235: 117–119

85   Snyder DS, Unanue ER (1982) Corticosteroids inhibit murine macrophage Ia expression and interleukin 1 production. *J Immunol* 129: 1803–1807

86   Lee SW, Tsou AP, Chan H, Thomas J, Petrie K, Eugui EM, Allison AC (1988) Gluco-corticoids selectively inhibit the transcription of the interleukin 1 beta decrease the sta-bility of interleukin 1 beta mRNA. *Proc Natl Acad Sci USA* 85: 1204–1208

87   Auphan N, Didonato JA, Rosette C, Helmberg A, Karin M (1995). Immunosuppression by glucocorticoids: inhibition of NF-κB activity through induction of Iκ synthesis. *Sci-ence* 270: 286–290

88   Scheinman RI, Gogswell PC, Lofquist AK, Baldwin Jr AS (1995) Role of transcription-al activation of 1κBα in mediation of immunosuppression by glucocorticoids. *Science* 270: 283–286

89   Siminoski K, Murphy RA, Rennert P, Heinrich G (1987) Cortisone, testosterone, and aldosterone reduce levels of nerve growth factor messenger ribonucleic acid in L-929 fibroblasts. *Endocrinol* 121: 1432–1437

90   Lindholm D, Hengerer B, Heumann R, Caroll P, Thoenen H (1990) Glucocorticoid hor-mones negatively regulate nerve growth expression *in vivo* and in cultured rat fibrob-lasts. *Eur J Neurosci* 2: 795–801

91   Rome LH, Lands WEM (1975) Structural requirements for time-dependent inhibition of prostaglandin biosynthesis by anti-inflammatory drugs. *Proc Natl Acad Sci USA* 72: 4863–4865

92   Friedman WJ, Larkfors L, Ayer-Lelievre C, Ebendal T, Olsson L, Persson H (1990) Reg-ulation of nerve growth factor expression by inflammatory mediators in hippocampal cultures. *J Neurosci Res* 27: 374–382

93   Salmon JA, Simmons PM, Moncada S (1983) The effects of BW755C and other anti-inflammatory drugs on eicosanoid concentrations and leukocyte accumulation in experimentally-induced acute inflammation. *J Pharm Pharmacol* 35: 808–813

94   Vane JR, Mitchell JA, Appleton I, Tomlinson A, Bishop-Bailey D, Croxtall J, Willough-by DA (1994) Inducible isoforms of cyclooxygenase and nitric-oxide synthase in inflam-mation. *Proc Natl Acad Sci USA* 91: 2046–2050

95   Maier JAM, Hlas T, Maciag T (1990) Cyclooxygenase is an immediate early gene induced by interleukin-1 in human endothelial cells. *J Biol Chem* 265: 10805–10808

96   Mitchell JA, Akarasereenont P, Themermann C, Flower RJ, Vane JR (1993) Selectivity

of non steroidal antiinflammatory drugs are inhibitors of constitutive and inducible cyclogenase. *Proc Natl Acad Sci USA* 90: 11693–11697

97 Masferrer JZ, Seibert K, Zweifel B, Needleman P (1992) Endogenous glucocorticoids regulate an inducible cyclooxygenase enzyme. *Proc Natl Acad Sci USA* 89: 3917–3921

98 Vassalli P (1992) The pathophysiology of tumor necrosis factors. *Ann Rev Immunol* 10: 411–452

99 Di Giovine FS, Malawista SE, Thornton E, Duff GW (1991) Urate crystals stimulate production of tumor necrosis factor alpha from human blood monocytes and synovial cells. Cytokine mRNA and protein kinetics, and cellular distribution. *J Clin Invest* 87: 1375–1381

100 Vilcek J, Lee TH (1991) Tumor necrosis factor. New insights into the molecular mechanisms of its multiple actions. *J Biol Chem* 266: 7313–7316

101 Zhang Y, Ramos BF, Jakschik B, Baganoff MP, Deppeler CL, Meyer DM, Widomski DL, Fretland DJ, Bolanowski MA (1995) Interleukin 8 and mast cell-generated tumor necrosis factor-alpha in neutrophil recruitment. *Inflammation* 19: 119–132

102 Issekutz AC, Meager A, Otterness I, Issekutz TB (1994) The role of tumour necrosis factor-alpha and IL-1 in polymorphoneclear leucocyte and T lymphocyte recruitment to joint inflammation in adjuvant arthritis. *Clin Exp Immunol* 97: 25–32

103 Lukacs NW, Strieter RM, Chensue SW, Widmer M, Kunkel SL (1995) TNF-alpha mediates recruitment of neutrophils and eosinophils during airway inflammation. *J Immunol* 154: 5411–5417

104 Hasko G, Elenkov IJ, Kvetan V & Vizi ES (1995) Differential effect of selective block of alpha 2-adrenoreceptors on plasma levels of tumour necrosis factor-alpha, interleukin-6 and corticosterone induced by bacterial lipopolysaccharide in mice. *J Endocrinol* 144: 457–462

105 Piguet PF, Grau GE, Hauser C, Vassalli P (1991) Tumor necrosis factor is a critical mediator in hapten induced irritant and contact hypersensitivity reactions. *J Exp Med* 173: 673–679

106 Sekut L, Menius JAJ, Brackeen MF, Connolly KM (1994) Evaluation of the significance of elevated levels of systemic and localized tumor necrosis factor in different animal models of inflammation. *J Lab Clin Med* 124: 813–820

107 Lessalauer W, Tabuchi H, Gentz R, Brockhaus M, Schlaeger EJ, Grau G, Piguet PF, Pointaire P, Vassalli P, Loetscher H (1991) Recombinant soluble tumor necrosis factor receptor proteins protect mice from lipopolysaccharide-induced lethality. *Eur J Immunol* 21: 2883–2886

108 Cooper AL, Brouwer S, Turnbull AV, Luheshi GN, Hopkins SJ, Kunkel SL, Rothwell NJ (1994) Tumor necrosis factor-alpha and fever after peripheral inflammation in the rat. *Am J Physiol* 267: R1431–R1436

109 Rankin EC, Choy EH, Kassimos D, Kingsley GH, Sopwith AM, Isenberg DA, Panayi GS (1995) The therapeutic effects of an engineered human anti-tumour necrosis factor alpha antibody (CDP571) in rheumatoid arthritis. *Br J Rheumatol* 34: 334–342

110 Williams RO, Ghrayeb J, Feldmann M, Maini RN (1995) Successful therapy of colla-

127

gen-induced arthritis with TNF receptor-IgG fusion protein and combination with anti-CD4. *Immunol* 84: 433–439

111 Cunha FQ, Poole S, Lorenzetti BB, Ferreira SH (1992) The pivotal role of tumour necrosis factor alpha in the development of inflammatory hyperalgesia. *Br J Pharmacol* 107: 660–664

112 Watkins LR, Goehler LE, Relton J, Brewer MT, Maier SF (1995) Mechanisms of tumor necrosis factor-alpha (TNF-alpha) hyperalgesia. *Brain Res*, 692: 244–250

113 Ferreira SH, Lorenzetti BB, Poole S (1993) Bradykinin initiates cytokine-mediated inflammatory hyperalgesia. *Br J Pharmacol* 110: 1227–1231

114 Woolf CJ, Allchorne A, Safieh-Garabedian B, Poole S (1997) Cytokines, nerve growth factor and inflammatory hyperalgesia: the contribution of tumour necrosis factor α. *Br J Pharmacol* 121: 417–424

115 Woolf CJ, MA Q-P, Allchorne A, Poole S (1996) Peripheral cell types contributing to the hyperalgesic action of nerve growth factor in inflammation. *J Neurosci* 16: 2716–2723

116 Neumann S, Doubell TP, Leslie TA, Woolf CJ (1996) Inflammatory pain hypersensitivity mediated by phenotypic switch in myelinated primary sensory neurones. *Nature* 384: 360–364

117 Lotz M, Moats T, Villiger PM (1992) Leukemia inhibitory factor is expressed in cartilage and synovium and can contribute to the pathogenesis of arthritis. *J Clin Invest* 90: 888–896

118 Waring P, Wycherley K, Cary D, Nicola N, Metcalf D (1992) Leukemia inhibitory factor levels are elevated in septic shock and various inflammatory body fluids. *J Clin Invest* 90: 2031–2037

119 Szepietowski JC, McKenzie RC, Keohane SG, Walker C, Aldridge RD, Hunter JA (1997) Leukemia inhibitory factor: induction in the early phase of allergic contact dermatitis. *Contact Dermatitis* 36: 21–25

120 Alexander HR, Billingsley KG, Block MI, Fraker DL (1994) D-factor/leukemmia inhibitory factor: evidence for its role as a mediator in acute and chronic inflammatory disease. *Cytokine* 6: 589–596

121 Brown MA, Metcalf D, Gough NM (1994) Leukaemia inhibitory factor and interleukin 6 are expressed at very low levels in the normal adult mouse and are induced by inflammation. *Cytokine* 6: 300–309

122 Ulich TR, Fann M-J, Patterson PH, Williams JH, Samal B, Del Castillo J, Yin S, Guo K, Remick DG (1994) Intrathecal injection of LPS and cytokines. V. LPS induces expression of LIF and LIF inhibits acute inflammation. *Amer Physiol Soc* 267: 442–446

123 Heyman D, L'Her E, Nguyen J-M, Raher S, Canfrere I, Coupey L, Fixe P, Chailleux S, De Grotte D, Praloran V, Godard A (1996) Leukemia inhibitory factor (LIF) production in pleural effusions: comparision with production of IL-4, IL-8, IL-10 and macrophage-colony stimulating factor (M-CSF). *Cytokine* 8: 416

124 Benigni F, Fantuzzi G, Sacco S, Sironi M, Pozzi P, Dinarello CA, Sipe JD, Poli V, Cappelletti M, Paonessa G et al (1996) Six different cytokines that share GP130 as a receptor subunit, induce serum amyloid A and potentiate the induction of interleukin-6 and

the activation of the hypothalamus-pituitary-adrenal axis by interleukin-1. *Blood* 87: 1851–1854

125 Weinhold B, Ruther U (1997) Interleukin-6-dependent and -independent regulation of the human C-reactive protein gene. *Biochem J* 327: 425–429

126 Ryffel B (1993) Pathology induced by leukemia inhibitory factor. *Int Rev Exp Pathol* 34: 69–72

127 Villiger PM, Geng Y, Lotz M (1993) Induction of cytokine expression by leukemia inhibitory factor. *J Clin Invest* 91: 1575–1581

128 Paglia D, Kondo S, Ng K-M, Sauder DN, McKenzie RC (1996) Leukemia inhibitory factor is expressed by normal human keratinocytes *in vitro* and *in vivo*. *Br J Dermatol* 134: 817–823

129 Block MI, Berg M, McNamara MJ, Norton JA, Fraker DL, Alexander HR (1993) Passive immunization of mice against D factor blocks lethality and cytokine release during endotoxemia. *J Exp Med* 178: 1085–1090

130 Carroll GJ, Bell MC, Chapman HM, Mills JN, Robinson WF (1995) Leukemia inhibitory factor induces leukocyte infiltration and cartilage proteoglycan degradation in goat joints. *J Interferon Cytokine Res* 15: 567–573

131 McKenzie RC, Paglia D, Kondo S, Sauder DN (1996) A novel endogenous mediator of cutaneous inflammation: leukemia inhibitory factor. *Acta Derm Venerol (Stockh)* 76: 111–114

132 Patterson PH (1994) Leukemia inhibitory factor, a cytokine at the interface between neurobiology and immunology. *Proc Natl Acad Sci USA* 91: 7833–7835

133 Kurek JB, Austin L, Cheema SS, Bartlett PF, Murphy M (1996) Up-regulation of leukemia inhibitory factor and interleukin-6 in transected sciatic nerve and muscle following denervation. *Neuromusc Disorders* 6: 105–114

134 Banner LR, Moayeri NN, Patterson PH (1997) Leukemia inhibitory factor is expressed in astrocytes following cortical injury. *Exp Neurol* 147: 1–9

135 Rao MS, Sun Y, Escrary JL, Perreau J, Tresser S, Patterson PH, Zigmond RE, Brulet P, Landes SL (1993) Leukemia inhibitory factor mediates an injury response but not a target-directed developmental transmitter switch in sympathetic neurons. *Neuron* 11: 1175–1185

136 Corness J, Shi T-J, Xu Z-Q, Brulet P, Hokfelt T (1996) Influence of leukemia inhibitory factor on galanin/GMAP and neuropeptide Y expression in mouse primary sensory neurons after axotomy. *Exp Brain Res* 112: 79–88

137 Sun Y, Zigmond RE (1996) Leukemia inhibitory factor induced in the sciatic nerve after axotomy is involved in the induction of galanin in sensory neurons. *Eur J Neurosci* 8: 2213–2220

138 Akita S, Malkin J, Melmed S (1996) Disrupted murine leukemia inhibitory factor (LIF) gene attenuates adrenocorticotropic hormone (ACTH) secretion. *Endocrinol* 137: 3140–3143

139 Ray DW, Ren SG, Melmed S (1996) Leukemia inhibitory factor (LIF) stimulates proop-

iomelanocortin (POMC) expression in a corticotroph cell lline. Role of STAT pathway. *J Clin Invest* 97: 1852–1859

140 Shimon I, Yan X, Ray DW, Melmed S (1997) Cytokine-dependent gp130 receptor sub-unit regulates human fetal pituitary adrenocorticotropin hormone and growth hormone secretion. *J Clin Invest* 100: 357–363

141 Banner LR, Patterson, P, Allchorne A, Poole S, Woolf, CJ (1998) *J Neurosci* 18: 5456–5462

142 Barnes PJ (1996) Neuroeffector mechanisms: the interface between inflammation and neuronal responses. *J Allergy Clin Immunol* 98: S73–81

143 Lynn B, Schutterle S, Pierau FK (1996) The vasodilator component of neurogenic inflammation is caused by a special subclass of heat-sensitive nociceptors in the skin of the pig. *J Physiol (Lond)* 494: 587–593

144 Thompson SWN, Dray A, Urban L (1996) Leukemia inhibitory factor induces mechan-ical allodynia but not thermal hyperalgesia in the juvenile rat. *Neurosci* 71: 1091–1094

145 Stahl N, Yancopoulos GD (1994) The tripartite CNRF receptor complex: activation and signaling involves components shared with other cytokines. *J Neurobiol* 25: 1454–1466

146 Dinarello CA (1996) Biologic basis for interleukin-1 in disease. *Blood* 87: 2095–2147

147 Campbell IK, Waring P, Novak U, Hamilton JA (1993) Production of leukemia inhibito-ry factor by human articular chondrocytes and cartilage in response to interleukin-1 and tumor necrosis factor alpha. *Arthritis Rheum* 36: 790–794

148 Handwerker HO, Reeh PW (1991) Pain and inflammation. In: MR Bond, JE Charlton, CE Wolf (eds): *Proceedings of the VIth World Congress on Pain.* Elsevier, Amsterdam, 59–70

149 Levine JD, Taiwo YO (1994) Inflammatory pain. In: PD Wall, R Melzack (eds): *Text-book of pain,* 3rd ed. Churchill Livingstone, Edinburgh, 45–56

150 Woolf CJ, Thompson SWN (1991) The induction and maintenance of central sensitiza-tion is dependent on N-methyl-D-aspartic acid receptor activation; implications for the treatment of post-injury pain hypersensitivity states. *Pain* 44: 293–299

151 Ma Q-P, Woolf CJ (1995) Involvement of neurokinin receptors in the induction but not the maintenance of mechanical allodynia in the rat flexor motoneurones. *J Physiol (Lond)* 486.3: 769–777

152 Klein R, Jing S, Nanduri V, O'Rourke E, Barbacid M (1991) The *trk* proto-oncogene encodes a receptor for nerve growth factor. *Cell* 65: 189–197

153 Kaplan DR, Hempstead BL, Martin-Zanca D, Chao MV, Parada LF (1991a) The *trk* proto-oncogene product: a signal transducing receptor for nerve growth factor. *Science* 252: 554–558

154 Lomen-Hoerth C, Shooter EM (1995) Widespread neurotrophin receptor expression in the immune system and other nonneuronal rat tissues. *J Neurochem* 64: 1780–1789

155 Wright DE, Snider WD (1995) Neurotrophin receptor mRNA expression defines dis-tinct populations of neurons in rat dorsal root ganglia. *J Comp Neurol* 351: 329–338

156 Averill S, McMahon SB, Clary DO, Reichardt LF, Priestley JV (1995) Immunocyto-

chemical localization of *trkA* receptors in chemically identified subgroups of adult rat sensory neurons. *Eur J Neurosci* 7: 1484–1494

157 Crowley C, Spencer S, Nishimura M, Chen KS, Pitts Meek S, Armanini MP, Ling LH, McMahon SB, Shelton DL, Levinson AD (1994) Mice laking nerve growth factor display perinatal loss of sensory and sympathetic neurons yet develop basal forebrain cholinergic neurons. *Cell* 76(6): 1001–1011

158 Otten U (1991) Nerve growth factor: A signalling protein between the nervous and the immune system. In: AI Basbaum, J-M Besson (eds): T*owards a new pharmacotherapy of pain*. John Wiley & Sons, Chichester, 353–363

159 Matsuda H, Switzer J, Coughlin MD, Bienenstock J, Denburg JA (1988) Human basophilic cell differentiation promoted by 2.5S nerve growth factor. *Int Arch Allergy Appl Immunol* 86: 453–457

160 Kannan Y, Matsuda H, Ushio H, Kawamoto K, Shimada Y (1993) Murine granulocyte-macrophage and mast cell colony formation promoted by nerve growth factor. *Int Arch Allergy Immunol* 102: 362–367

161 Melamed I, Turner CE, Aktories K, Kaplan DR, Gelfand EW (1995) Nerve growth factor triggers microfilament assembly and paxillin phosphorylation in human B lymphocytes. *J Exp Med* 181(3): 1071–1079

162 Marshall JS, Bienenstock J (1994) The role of mast cells in inflammatory reactions of the airways, skin and intestine. *Curr Opin Immunol* 6: 853–859

163 Horigome K, Bullock ED, Johnson EMJ (1994) Effects of nerve growth factor on rat peritoneal mast cells. Survival promotion and immediate-early gene induction. *J Biol Chem* 269: 2695–2702

164 Marshall JS, Stead RH, McSharry C, Nielsen L, Bienenstock J (1990) The role of mast cell degranulation products in mast cell hyperplasia. I Mechanism of action of nerve growth factor. *J Immunol* 144: 1886–1892

165 Schwartz LB (1994) Mast cells: function and contents. *Curr Opin Immunol* 6: 91–97

166 Coderre TJ, Basbaum AI, Levine JD (1989) Neural control of vascular permeability: interactions between primary afferents, mast cells, and sympathetic efferents. *J Neurophysiol* 62: 48–58

167 Levi-Montalcini R (1987) The nerve growth factor: thirty-five years later. *EMBO J* 6: 1145–1154

168 Davis BM, Lewin GR, Mendell LM, Jones ME, Albers KM (1993) Altered expression of nerve growth factor in the skin of transgenic mice leads to profound changes in response to mechanical stimuli. *Neurosci* 56: 789–795

169 Andreev NY, Dimitrieva N, Koltzenburg M, McMahon SB (1995) Peripheral administration of nerve growth factor in the adult rat produces a thermal hyperalgesia that requires the presence of sympathetic postganglionic neurones. *Pain* 63: 109–115

170 Levine JD, Taiwo YO, Collins SD, Tam JK (1986) Noradrenaline hyperalgesia is mediated through interaction with sympathetic postganglionic neurone terminals rather than activation of primary afferent nociceptors. *Nature* 323: 158–160

171 Nakamura M, Ferreira SH (1987) A peripheral sympathetic component in inflammatory hyperalgesia. *Eur J Pharmacol* 135: 145–153

172 Perrot S, Attal N, Ardid D, Guilbaud G (1994) Are mechanical and clod allodynia in monineuropathic and arthritic rats relieved by systemic treatment with calcitonin or guanethidine. *Pain* 52(1): 41–47

173 Lam FY, Ferrell WR (1991) Neurogenic component of different models of acute inflammation in the rat knee joint. *Ann Rheum Dis* 50: 747–751

174 Sluka KA, Lawand NB, Westlund KN (1994) Joint inflammation is reduced by dorsal rhizotomy and not by sympathectomy or spinal cord transection. *Ann Rheum Dis* 53: 309–314

175 Kaplan DR, Stephens RM (1994) Neurotrophin signal transduction by the *trk* receptor. *J Neurobiol* 25(11): 1404–1417

176 Toledo-Aral JJ, Brehm P, Halegoua S, Mandel G (1995) A single pulse of nerve growth factor triggers long-term neuronal excitability through sodium channel gene induction. *Neuron* 14: 607–611

177 Lembeck F, Donnerer J, Tsuchiya M, Nagahisa A (1992) The non-peptide tachykinin antagonist, CP-96,345, is a potent inhibitor of neurogenic inflammation. *Br J Pharmacol* 105(3): 527–530

178 Woolf CJ (1983) Evidence for a central component of post-injury pain hypersensitivity. *Nature* 306: 686–688

179 Woolf CJ, Wall PD (1986) The relative effectiveness of C primary afferent fibres of different origins in evoking a prolonged facilitation of the flexor reflex in the rat. *J Neurosci* 6: 1433–1443

Hyperalgesic actions of cytokines on peripheral nerves

Robert R. Myers[1,2], Rochelle Wagner[1] and Linda S. Sorkin[1]

VA Medical Center and the University of California, San Diego, Departments of Anesthesiology[1] and Pathology (Neuropathology)[2], 9500 Gilman Drive, La Jolla, CA 92093-0629, USA

Introduction

The relationship between nerve injury and pain is pervasive in medicine, being both a simple, common experience and an important diagnostic tool. Acute trauma to a nerve is almost always painful and has been experienced by many people in association with sports and workplace activities. In these cases, injuries occur usually because of nerve stretching or compression, damaging sensory axons that will then degenerate and regenerate. If the nerve is not transected and the Schwann cell basal lamina of the nerve fiber is left intact, the prognosis for recovery is good since regenerating axons are appropriately guided to the original target tissue. If neuropathic pain states do not develop, acute pain will normally resolve during the period of axonal regeneration, which begins within about a week after nerve injury and the start of nerve fiber degeneration. Misguided regeneration that produces a neuroma in continuity or, more often, a neuroma at the severed end of the nerve bundle, can be persistently painful because of the sensitivity of the undifferentiated free nerve endings to mechanical pressure and chemical stimuli. Another example is the subchronic low back pain syndrome caused by nerve root compression and chemical irritation secondary to herniated spinal discs. This and other forms of subchronic nerve injury caused by repeated physical or chemical irritation become more problematic in terms of predicting the duration of pain. In these cases, there is often ongoing and intermixed degeneration and regeneration that not only produces acute pain but can also lead to facilitated central processing of peripheral nociceptive signals and chronic pain states. Chronic nerve injuries can be more painful still, but may also be so severe or widespread that nociceptive axons and first-order sensory neurons in the dorsal root ganglia are permanently damaged so that peripheral stimuli are not meaningfully transduced. Severe diabetic neuropathy fits this description if it progresses through states of paresthesia, hyperalgesia, hypoalgesia, and anesthesia. Other causes of complete nerve injury such as iatrogenic transection of

Cytokines and Pain, edited by Linda R. Watkins and Steven F. Maier
© 1999 Birkhäuser Verlag Basel/Switzerland

peripheral nerves during limb amputation may lead to deafferentation syndromes in which phantom pain is prevalent, although some models of deafferentation imply that phantom pain may be associated with regeneration [1].

The classification of traumatic nerve injuries and other peripheral neuropathies has been useful in establishing common mechanisms of injury and the expected clinical pain syndromes [2]. To gain insight into the relationship between abnormal nerve morphology and pain, several authors have used biopsied and post-mortem samples of human tissue to correlate with the corresponding clinical measures of pain [3–5]. As reviewed by Scadding [2], the results suggest that pain is not related only to changes in fiber size distribution, but rather to neuropathies in which there is rapid axonal degeneration. While neuropathies involving small fibers are often painful, the simultaneous expression of degenerative and regenerative events appears to be a more important factor associated with pain. It is also recognized that ischemia can exacerbate paresthesia and pain following peripheral nerve damage as well as cause axonal degeneration if it is severe or prolonged. These general conclusions, however, fail to account for all the clinical findings linking nerve injury and pain, and may be further complicated by such factors as sympathetically-mediated pain seen sometimes in association with traumatic mononeuropathies and by psychosocial factors. To date, no unifying hypothesis has been fully supported by the accumulated evidence available from human studies.

Animal studies hold the key to further understanding of painful neuropathies. Animal studies in both invertebrates and vertebrates have reinforced the insights from clinical experience and extended them by providing for controlled temporal investigations and experimental therapy. In combination with standard tests for allodynia [6] and newly developed techniques for testing thermal escape responses [7], it has been demonstrated that a behavioral hyperalgesia and/or mechanical allodynia can be modeled in the rodent with partial nerve injury [8–10]. The chronic constriction injury (CCI) model of neuropathic pain [8] has been particularly useful in exploring the role of focal nerve ischemia and axonal (Wallerian) degeneration of nerve fibers in the pathogenesis of neuropathic pain states [11–13]. CCI neuropathy develops within days after placing loose chromic gut ligatures around the sciatic nerve. The ligatures are tied loosely such that epineurial blood vessels are constricted, reducing endoneurial blood flow initially by approximately 50 percent [11]. Rapid development of endoneurial edema increases the fascicular area and effectively tightens the ligatures [14–15]. This physical injury, in combination with the inflammatory insult caused by the chromic gut ligatures, produces severe Wallerian degeneration and hyperalgesia (Figs. 1, 2).

We have hypothesized that the initial neuropathological events at the site of peripheral nerve injury are important in initiating the complex cascade of changes in proximal sensory function that define neuropathic pain states. Early evidence in support of the hypothesis [16] showed that blockade of retrograde axonal transport by colchicine applied topically to nerve between the peripheral nerve injury and dorsal root ganglia (DRG) eliminated the expected hyperalgesia. While colchicine blocked the retrograde transport of target-derived factors to the DRG, it also blocked anterograde transport of new sodium channels to regenerating axonal sprouts. Our pathological analyses suggest that while the accumulation of sodium channels in axonal sprouts of neuromas may be important in potentiating the neuropathic pain state, other factors are probably more important in the development of hyperalgesia. These electrophysiological and chemical factors are generated by the injury or are released at the injury site before sodium channel production is upregulated. Target-derived chemical factors include cytokines and proteolytic products of activated Schwann cells and macrophages whose chemical activities cause disruption of nerve fibers and upregulation of neurotrophic factors.

Cytokines orchestrate the pathological, and arguably the pathophysiological, events at the site of experimental nerve injury and can be considered as the unifying factor(s) that control the development of neuropathic pain. Cytokine synthesis is directly related to the temporal course of the many events noted to be involved in observations of neuropathic pain. These events can be viewed as neuroimmunological responses to tissue injury and can be modulated with anti-inflammatory cytokine therapy to reduce both nerve injury and pain. This extension of our understanding of neuropathological processes is the general consequence of improved understanding of cytokine actions and focused experiments in rodent models of painful nerve injury. It is reasonable to expect that this knowledge can be used in support of new therapeutic strategies and, in fact, preliminary experiments reviewed below are demonstrating this utility.

Pathogenesis of proinflammatory nerve injury

In a certain sense, the response to all nerve injuries is inflammatory in nature in that the principal cellular mediators of nerve degeneration are immune cells and macrophages recruited to the injury site in response to immunological signals thought to be mediated by proinflammatory cytokines. Following nerve injury, there is a complex series of events causing pain and structural damage to peripheral axons and their afferent cell bodies. The events are intertwined and graded in scale to produce responses appropriate to the stimulus. Studies in the marine invertebrate *Aplysia californica* suggest that there are early, intermediate, and late signals from the site of nerve injury that combine to alter gene expression in the pedal ganglia and regulate the machinery for the synthesis and processing of proteins required for regeneration and compensatory plasticity of the cell body [17]. Early events include the electrophysiological "injury discharge" which alters the neuronal influx of calcium to activate protein kinases such as calmodulin (CaM) kinase II and IV, protein kinases A and C, and mitogen-associated protein (MAP) kinase which regulate transcription factors. Intermediate signals are conveyed by retrograde transport and can

135

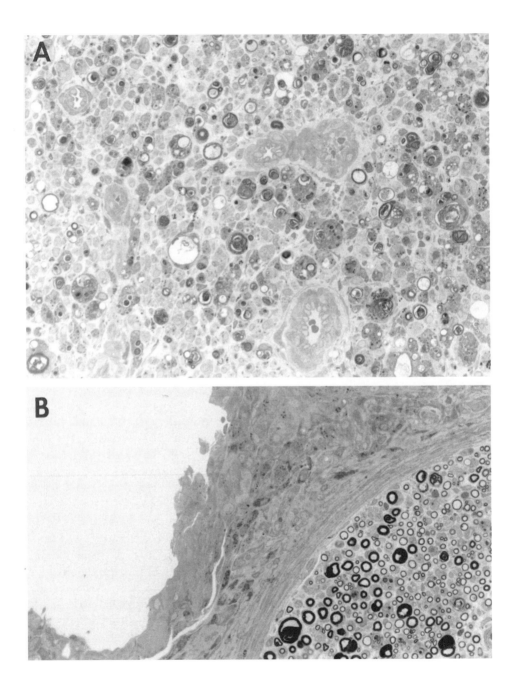

either repress or promote transcription factors for regeneration [18, 19]. The transcription factor targets such as c-Jun and NF-kB exert control over the synthesis of proteins necessary for regeneration and processing of nociceptive information. Cytokines represent signals generated from hours to weeks after nerve injury and thus span the intermediate and late time frames associated with signal transduction events. Proinflammatory cytokines increase the sensitivity of all peripheral neural structures and their afferent cell bodies, causing hyperalgesia and the development of neuropathic pain states [20, 21]. The full complement of these early, intermediate and late processes is invoked in the pathogenesis of neuropathic pain with perhaps upregulation of proinflammatory cytokine events being the single most important and treatable factor linked to the development of chronic pain.

With respect to the cytokine events in this multiphase response to nerve injury, there is also a chemical hierarchy that has been postulated to occur. For example, the release of substance P (sP) from peripheral sensory terminals and injured axons contributes to neurogenic inflammation by inducing vasodilatation, plasma extravasation and mast cell degranulation [22]. The granular contents of mast cells are known to contain tumor necrosis factor α (TNFα), interleukins, granulocyte-macrophage-colony stimulation factor (GM-CSF), chemotactic agents, and nerve growth factor (NGF) [23]. These cytokine factors then influence the sequence of events associated with nerve degeneration that are described in the pathological literature as Wallerian degeneration. Thus, it may be through this initial interaction with neuropeptides that cytokines become involved in the inflammatory process associated with nerve injury and pain.

Figure 1
Wallerian degeneration of endoneurial nerve fibers is the principal pathological finding in the chronic constriction injury (CCI) neuropathy. Nerve degeneration begins within hours after placement of the CCI ligatures as a response to endoneurial ischemia and the inflammatory challenge of the ligatures. Endoneurial edema is an early finding in the pathology of the neuropathy. Degeneration of nerve fibers (myelin and axons) is initiated by activated Schwann cells and is later reinforced by macrophages recruited to the injury site from the systemic circulation. (A) Severe Wallerian degeneration is seen in this 1-µm-thick, plastic-embedded section of rat sciatic nerve seven days after CCI. Phagocytic macrophages and Schwann cells are seen throughout the field. Endothelial cells are also severely affected by CCI and are seen here to be swollen and lined with plasma cells. (B) Following Wallerian degeneration, regeneration of nerve fibers occur. This section is from a rat 23 days after CCI and demonstrates extensive remyelination as indicated by thinly myelinated axons. Axonal sprouts are not seen at this magnification. The hole in the upper left is the remnant site of a CCI ligature. Paraphenylenediamine-stained, 1 µm plastic-embedded sections, 200× original magnification.

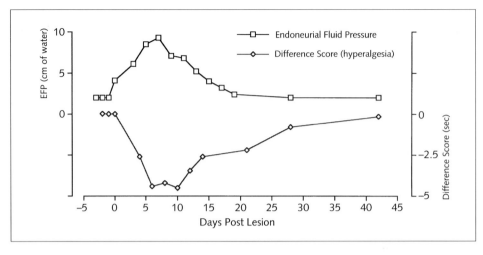

Figure 2
Thermal hyperalgesia associated with chronic constriction injury of rat sciatic nerve. As displayed in Figure 1, CCI produces a neuropathy involving substantial Wallerian degeneration of the adjacent nerve fibers and subsequent regeneration. These processes parallel the development and resolution of hyperalgesia. The upper curve represents changes in endoneurial fluid pressure (EFP) in Wallerian degeneration and has a normal value of 2 cm H_2O. EFP increases during the active phase of Wallerian degeneration and returns to normal during the period of regeneration. EFP reflects the increased endoneurial space occupied by macrophages and mitotic Schwann cells, and by edema associated with changes in the permeability of the blood-nerve barrier. Hyperalgesia to thermal stimuli (bottom curve) is reflected as a negative difference score and is derived by comparing the latency to withdrawal of the control and experimental footpads from a focal heat stimuli. The period of maximal hyperalgesia corresponds to the peak period of macrophage activity in Wallerian degeneration.

Role of Wallerian degeneration in nerve injury and pain

Crushing or transecting a peripheral nerve begins a process of degeneration which extends from the injury site to the distal receptor in a proximodistal direction; several millimeters of the nerve proximal to the injury site may also degenerate. If the injury occurs too close to the cell body, the cell and its processes will die; otherwise, regeneration of the nerve fiber will ensue after degeneration. Incomplete nerve injuries involving axons also produce similar forms of pathological change in the affected fibers. The degeneration process is known as Wallerian degeneration and was first described by Augustus Waller in 1850 following nerve transection. The axoplasm gradually disintegrates, and the axolemma fragments with its contents undergoing granular dissolution. During this time the myelin sheath of the Schwann cell may remain intact, but it then forms lamellar ovoids surrounded by Schwann cell cytoplasm (Fig. 3). Schwann cells may phagocytose myelin debris, and this process is assisted by hematogenously derived macrophages (Fig. 3). This is the process that is most closely correlated with the development of hyperalgesia in nerve-injured animals. We confirmed this clinical observation after a series of experiments designed to compare a range of experimental neuropathies with the magnitude and duration of the associated sensory deficit [11]. The nerve injury models included mild ischemia resulting in selective damage to Schwann cells and demyelination, severe ischemic injury producing moderate degrees of Wallerian degeneration, chronic inflammatory constriction injury producing severe Wallerian degeneration, and crush injury. Crush injury to all nerve fibers produced a sensory block while the other forms of injury produced graded degrees of hyperalgesia ranging from mild hyperalgesia associated with ischemic injuries producing demyelination to severe and protracted hyperalgesia associated with severe Wallerian degeneration after chronic constriction nerve injury with inflammation-promoting sutures.

Wallerian degeneration is dependent on activity of macrophages recruited to the injury site [24, 25]. Following nerve injury, non-resident, hematogeneous macrophages invade the injury site, their numbers peaking during the intense period of phagocytic activity associated with Wallerian degeneration. Coincidentally, the peak in hyperalgesia parallels the invasion of macrophages [14]. Bruche and Friede [24] demonstrated that non-resident macrophages are the primary effector cell in Wallerian degeneration by showing that severed nerves did not degenerate when they were isolated in a Millipore chamber that excluded the entry of macrophages. Additional insights into the relationship between nerve degeneration and macrophage activity have been significantly advanced by the chance discovery of a mouse mutant (WLD) in which there is delayed recruitment of hematogeneous macrophages to the site of nerve injury [26, 27]. Although it has been shown that Wallerian degeneration can be inhibited by preventing the recruitment of macrophages with a monoclonal antibody against their complement type 3 receptor, this is apparently not the reason for delayed recruitment of macrophages to the injured nerve in WLD animals. Rather, there is a genetic defect that affects the required chemotactic signal from injured axons or Schwann cells [28]. Macrophage function, per se, is normal in WLD animals since macrophages respond appropriately to injuries outside the nervous system. Two research groups have now demonstrated that this delay in macrophage recruitment to the injury site and the consequent delayed Wallerian degeneration is associated with reduced neuropathic pain [29, 30]. Bisby and colleagues [31–33] show that both sensory and motor neuron axon regeneration is impaired in WLD mice, yet the initial cell body response to nerve injury is no different from that of normal mice. Associated with the delayed Wallerian degenera-

139

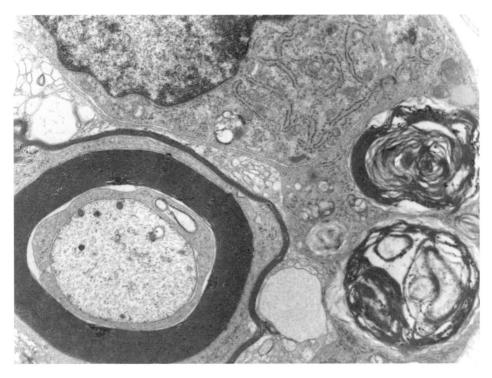

Figure 3
Macrophages are seen phagocytosing myelin and Schwann cell debris five days after chronic constriction injury to the rat sciatic nerve. Myelin splitting is a consequence of endoneurial TNF which targets the Schwann cell or its myelin sheath. Note that while the axon appears normal at this time point, severe demyelination may also affect the integrity of the axon, and that TNF may also directly target the axon. Macrophages can penetrate the basal lamina of activated Schwann cells to phagocytose the cell and its associated axon during the process of Wallerian degeneration. Electron micrograph stained with uranyl acetate and lead citrate, 16,000× original magnification.

tion, there is a delayed increase in NGF levels in the denervated distal stump. Finally, Ramer et al. [30] report that Wallerian degeneration is required for sympathetic sprouting into the DRG, suggesting that NGF mediates these structural changes that are thought to be important in neuropathic pain states [34].

We reasoned that cytokines or another product of macrophage activation was crucial in initiating the cascade of events leading to neuropathic pain states. Although all the mechanisms by which macrophages potentiate Wallerian degeneration are not known, it is thought that cytokine signaling and secretion of proteases play a central role. Activated macrophages show profound differences in membrane proteins and transcription that alter the synthesis, expression, and location of cell-bound and secretory proteins. Activated macrophages secrete components of the complement cascade, coagulation factors, proteases, hydrolases, interferons, TNF, interleukins and other cytokines [35] that directly influence the structure and function of both adjacent and distal tissues. For example, it is well known that the release of interleukin-1 (IL-1) from activated macrophages in the endoneurial space stimulates the synthesis of NGF by Schwann cells [36]; peripheral nerve regeneration is impeded in the presence of an IL-1 receptor antagonist and in WLD mice, as discussed above.

Thus, cytokines appear to be important communication links between key support cells in the endoneurium that control the endoneurial environment, the processes of Wallerian degeneration, and the production of trophic factors required for regeneration. The importance of understanding the complex relationships between macrophages, Schwann cells, and mast cells that function normally to regulate the immune reactions of nerve fibers to injury and foreign antibodies is heightened by their association with the pathogenesis of neuropathic pain.

IL-1 and TNF are accepted at the present time as being two of the earliest and most important cytokines produced by activated macrophages. As already mentioned, IL-1 stimulates Schwann cells to express nerve growth factor on their surfaces, and retrograde transport of NGF and its receptor from the nerve injury site is an important signal affecting the function of DRG neurons. A full discussion of NGF effects on peripheral nerve function and pain is contained elsewhere in this book. Our focus has been on the local effect of TNF in the pathogenesis of pain since early experiments demonstrated that blocking the macrophage production of this cytokine reduced the degree of expected nerve injury and pain in CCI neuropathy [37]. The remainder of this chapter focuses on our understanding of the role of TNF in neuropathic pain states.

Cytokine injuries to the PNS

The relationship between TNF and nerve injury has been of increasing interest since TNF was implicated in the pathogenesis of multiple sclerosis, HIV-associated neurological diseases, and peripheral demyelinating neuropathies [38–42]. Recent experimental *in vivo* studies in which human recombinant TNFα or TNFβ was injected into the sciatic nerve demonstrated a transient, dose-dependent, focal endoneurial inflammation that was followed by primary demyelination and axonal degeneration [43]. The findings were similar in nerves injected with either TNFα or TNFβ. There was evidence of leukocyte margination and transendothelial migration through vessels walls that were often thickened. Mononuclear cells in the subendothelial space, between the endothelium and peri-endothelial cells sometimes were so dense as to occlude this space, a finding that was directly related to the dose of TNF. In all the nerves injected, numerous polymorphonuclear leukocytes and macrophages were present within both the epineurium and endoneurium, and also between the layers of the perineurium. An earlier study [44] showed that nerves injected with different concentrations of TNF-enriched serum, recombinant TNF, and interferon showed axonal degeneration of 80% of the nerve fibers. In contrast, injection of lipopolysaccharide (LPS) produced little demyelination three days after injection. However, LPS would be expected to activate only the few resident macrophages present at the injection site, and at this early time-point there may not have been significant recruitment of hematogeneous macrophages to increase the cytokine concentration to levels obtained after direct injection of TNF. Our own work shows that TNF is capable of causing both demyelination and axonal injury. In fact, it is suggested that severe primary demyelinating neuropathies can be associated with axonal degeneration and that this is often the case seen clinically [45]. The pathogenesis of the injuries need not be different if macrophage products are involved. Perhaps the transition from demyelination to axonal degeneration relates only to an increase in the concentration and duration of exposure to the inflammatory cytokines and proteolytic enzymes. This hypothesis is contradicted however, by data that suggest a biphasic dose-response relationship between TNF and pathophysiological effect [46]. Nevertheless, to the extent that locally-generated TNF feeds back positively to activate additional recruited macrophages, there would be a mechanism to directly injure bystander axons.

Neuropathology of proinflammatory cytokines

Our work shows a progression in neuropathological change related to TNF dose. At low doses of TNF injection into rat sciatic nerve, there is substantial endoneurial edema accumulating in the subperineurial, perivascular and endoneurial spaces of the nerve bundle. The endoneurial edema separates individual nerve fibers that are normally tightly packed together. At doses in the range of 10 µl of a 2.5 pg/ml solution of murine recombinant TNF, extensive demyelination was observed along the injection tract where it was localized to a discrete area of the fascicle adjacent to the site of injection (Fig. 4). Study of tissue injected with a higher dose of TNF (25 pg/ml, 5 µl), showed extensive splitting of myelin lamellae which formed large vacuoles (Fig. 5) prior to demyelination. Schwann cell cytoplasm contained lipid debris consistent with their phagocytic role while macrophages invaded the tissue after three days to reinforce the phagocytic process. Activated fibroblasts were present in the endoneurium and there were reactive changes in endothelial cells. Occasional axons were seen to be undergoing Wallerian-like degeneration that was identifiable initially by swollen, dark-staining axons with intact myelin, and later by collapse of the axonal cylinder and progression of the degeneration distally.

142

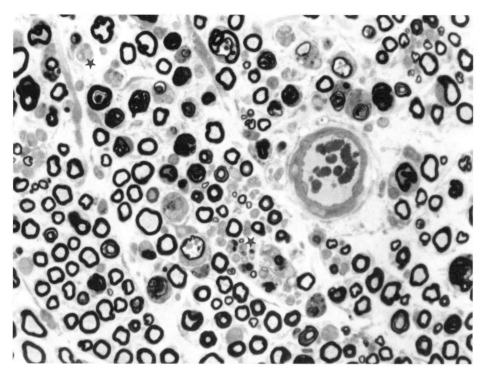

Figure 4
Transverse section of rat sciatic nerve three days after subperineurial injection of 10 μl TNF, 2.5 pg/ml. Note extensive endoneurial edema, reactive endothelial cells and demyelinated axons (star). Paraphenylenediamine-stained, 1 μm plastic-embedded section, 400× original magnification

These changes can also be seen in other inflammatory and ischemic neuropathies. Nukada and McMorran [47] demonstrate striking examples of intramyelinic edema following reperfusion nerve injury that exactly mimic the findings of low-dose TNF injection. Intramyelinic edema was due to splitting of the myelin lamellae at intraperiod lines. The pathology observed was predominantly perivascular and included demyelination in association with phagocytic cells and activated Schwann cells; vascular lesions included activated endothelial cells. Similar consequences are seen in an experimental neuritis model in the sciatic nerves of rats where the pathology has been linked to allodynia and hyperalgesia [48].

We observed that some normal Schwann cells have a basal immunoreactivity to TNF *in vivo* and that there is a significant increase in immunoreactivity during the degenerative phase of CCI neuropathy [49]. Using both immunohistochemistry staining for TNF protein in frozen-, paraffin-, and plastic-embedded sections, and

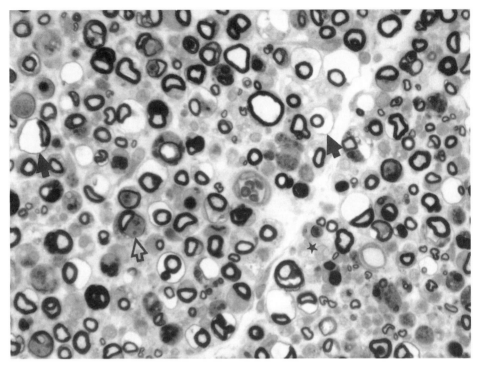

Figure 5

Transverse section of rat sciatic nerve injected with 5 μl TNF, 25 pg/ml. Note extensive demyelination (star), splitting of myelin lamellae (closed arrow) and hydropic and phagocytic Schwann cells (open arrow). Paraphenylenediamine-stained, 1 μm plastic-embedded section, 400× original magnification.

in situ hybridization for specific messenger RNA sequences in paraffin sections, we observed an increase in the number and density of Schwann cell cytoplasmic staining for both TNF protein and message (Figs. 6, 7). Other endoneurial cells immunopositive for TNF, and activated in CCI neuropathy, included endothelial cells, fibroblasts, and macrophages. Positive identification of cell type was facilitated by staining alternate tissue sections for glial fibrillary acidic protein, a known glial intermediate filament, and by structural analysis of cells in plastic-embedded tissue cut at 1 μm thickness. The initial increase in TNF immunoreactivity quantified 18 h after CCI injury was doubled by seven days, during the time of maximum macrophage involvement in the neuropathy. An increase in Schwann cell TNF immunoreactivity within 18 h following nerve injury [49] may serve several impor-

144

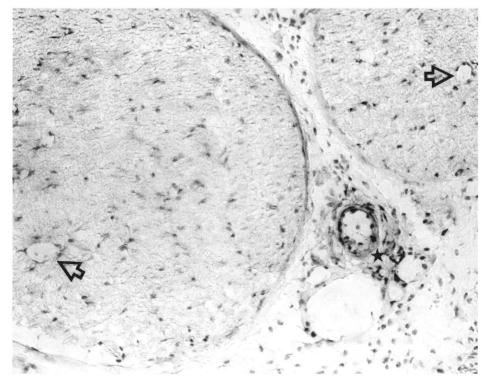

Figure 6
TNF immunohistochemistry in frozen section of rat sciatic nerve three days following chronic constriction injury. TNF-positive immune cells can be seen adjacent to the intraluminal wall of an epineurial vessel and in the adjacent perivascular space (star). TNF-positive cells can also be seen in the perivascular space of endoneurial blood vessels (arrow). Other TNF-positive cells within the endoneurium are Schwann cells, fibroblasts, and endothelial cells. 100× original magnification.

tant functions, including recruitment and activation of macrophages to the injury site as a second line of immunological defense, and facilitation of the phagocytic role of Schwann cells which contributes to the initial process of nerve fiber degeneration. This process is then extended and amplified by recruited macrophages which may in turn attack Schwann cells.

Another cytokine produced by Schwann cells is Interleukin-6 (IL-6). IL-6 mRNA is induced within 12 h of crush injury [50]. Using an immortal Schwann cell (iSC) culture, Bolin et al. [50] have shown that LPS, TNF, IL-1, and IL-6 induced IL-6

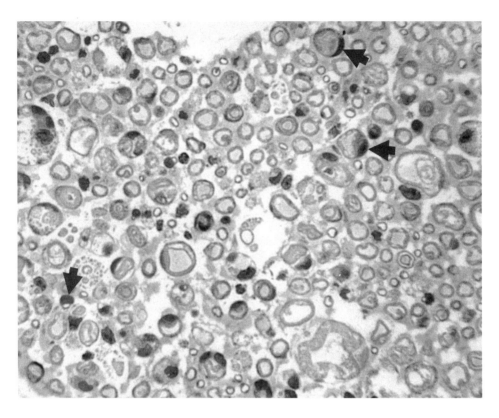

Figure 7
Resin-embedded rat sciatic nerve seven days after chronic constriction injury. One-micron-thick section immunostained for TNF-α. Note positive staining of Schwann cell cytoplasm (arrows). Macrophages, fibroblasts, and endothelial cells also stain positively for TNF during Wallerian degeneration. 400× original magnification.

mRNA production. There was expression of both the IL-6 receptor and the gp130 receptor component, suggesting an autocrine regulatory mechanism. In *in vivo* crush experiments, these authors demonstrated that IL-6 message was expressed distal to a crush injury and suggested that IL-6 may facilitate nerve regeneration through interaction with leukemia inhibitory factor (LIF). IL-6 and LIF, a member of the trophic family of cytokines, are multifunctional and related on the basis of their structural similarities and shared signal transducing receptor components [51]. Both are thought to act as trauma factors, but only LIF is a demonstrated neurotrophic factor for sensory neurons and is retrogradely transported to the cell body. The specific roles of IL-6 and LIF in abnormal sensation and pain are not yet established, but they might share a role with NGF in signaling nerve injury and modulating neuronal function.

Schwann cells are also of importance in that they are the first-order of immunological defense in peripheral nerves, along with the few resident macrophages seen in perivascular spaces. Schwann cells have a phagocytic role in neuropathy and express low levels of both major histocompatibility complex (MHC) class I and class II molecules.

TNF-induced pain

Murine recombinant TNF injected into Sprague-Dawley rat sciatic nerve produces a transient unilateral thermal hyperalgesia and mechanical allodynia [52]. Vehicle injection alone was without significant behavioral effect. In these studies, thermal hyperalgesia was quantified by the Hargreaves [7] technique and mechanical threshold by von Frey hairs [1]. Behavioral tests were made prior to injection of the experimental agent and for seven days following injection. The contralateral nerve was used for behavioral and histological control. Animals that received TNF displayed a statistically significant thermal hyperalgesia at days 1 and 3 post-injection compared with baseline values, as demonstrated by a decrease in the withdrawal latency of the affected foot (Fig. 8). This thermal hyperalgesia was somewhat variable in its onset, but lasted several days once established. Mechanical allodynia was demonstrated by a decrease in the withdrawal threshold from baseline values for TNF-injected animals throughout the week following injection (Fig. 9). While the duration of these abnormal behavioral responses were less than those associated with CCI neuropathy, the pathology was correspondingly reduced and there was not a robust macrophage response to the injection. Nevertheless, these data suggest that nociceptive behaviors commonly observed in models of experimental neuropathy can be mimicked by the injection of TNF into the endoneurium of the sciatic nerve and importantly connect the local distribution of a proinflammatory cytokine with the demonstration of pain-like behaviors in awake, intact animals.

One mechanism for these nociceptive effects of local TNF may have been revealed in recent experiments by Sorkin et al. [46]. In these experiments, topical application of TNF to the nerve trunk induced ectopic electrophysiological activity in single primary afferent nociceptive fibers consistent in frequency with that which is known to be associated with pain perception as well as central sensitization of the nociceptive system. This occurred within minutes of TNF application and without stimulation or sensitization of the peripheral sensory receptors located distally. However, when TNF was injected into the paw, these authors observed the electrophysiological and behavioral evidence of sensitization of peripheral nociceptive receptors reported by others [53] that was absent when TNF was applied midaxonally. These results suggest that TNF in the vicinity of the axon, independent of its

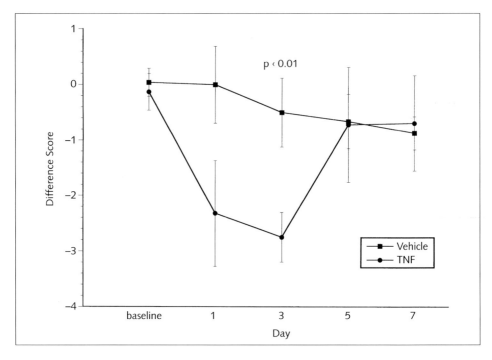

Figure 8
Thermal difference scores following endoneurial injection of TNF or vehicle.
Changes in the thermal difference score to paw heating as a measure of hyperalgesia fol-
lowing injection of TNF or vehicle in the experimental sciatic nerve or rats. Nerve injections
were of either 2.5 pg/ml TNF or 0.1% BSA/0.1M phosphate buffer (vehicle) in a 10 μl vol-
ume. TNF-injected animals displayed a significant decrease in thermal difference score when
compared with vehicle-injected animals at day 3 post-injection.

peripheral receptors, can lead to aberrant electrophysiological activity in nociceptive fibers. The effect was seen to be maximal between TNF concentrations of 0.001 to 0.01 ng/ml and absent at higher concentrations (Fig. 10) [46]. The TNF-mediated increase in electrophysiological activity was also more pronounced in C than in A-delta fibers.

Since the axons in these experiments were detached from their dorsal root ganglia, TNF application could not have resulted in transport or change in turnover of sodium or calcium channels known to be important in the spontaneous electro-physiological activity seen in other neuropathic pain and neuroma models [54]. While other less established mechanisms were also considered, we believed that one explanation is related to the unique biophysical properties of the active TNF trimer. Recent studies in cultured lymphoma cells [55] have revealed that the trimeric struc-

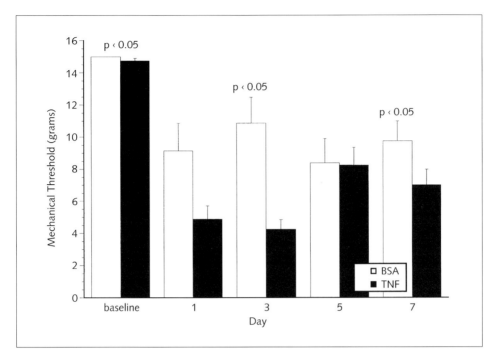

Figure 9
Mechanical threshold following endoneurial injection of TNF or vehicle.
Changes in the mechanical thresholds to withdrawal of the footpad in rats with injection of
TNF or vehicle in the ipsilateral sciatic nerve. Gram force scale derived from von Frey hair
stimulation. TNF-injected animals displayed a significant decrease in mechanical threshold
compared with vehicle-injected animals at days 1, 3, and 7 post-injection.

ture of bioactive TNF creates a pore throughout the entire length of its central axis and that after binding to its receptor, this structure is inserted into the cellular membrane. This process is enhanced by low pH [56]. These novel TNF channels are permeable to sodium ions in a oubain-independent manner, and are voltage-dependent [57]. Thus, if these results can be used to predict membrane events in isolated rat axons, sodium conductance would increase immediately upon repolarization and could induce axons to fire spontaneously at relatively high frequencies.

In summary, these data suggest a new mechanism by which injury to the axon can lead to neuropathic pain states. The local liberation of TNF from mast cells, Schwann cells, macrophages, and other cells at the site of nerve injury and the possible nearly instantaneous insertion of the TNF trimer into the axonal membrane could cause a voltage-dependent increase in sodium permeability. This process may

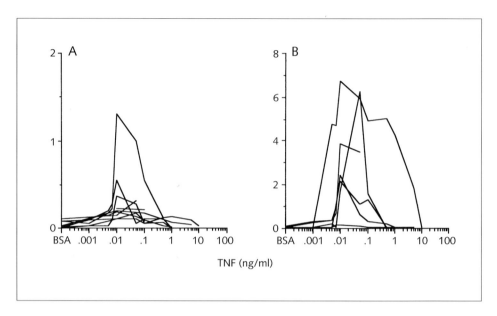

Figure 10
Sequential increases in concentration of TNF administered to a 4 mm length of rat sciatic nerve produced a U-shaped dose-response in each fiber. (A) Individual responses of seven myelinated Aδ fibers. (B) Responses of six unmyelinated C fibers. Bovine serum albumin (BSA), 0.1% in normal saline, was used for control and administered prior to TNF application.

then be potentiated several days later by the release of additional TNF and other cytokines from macrophages recruited to the injury site. High concentrations of TNF may activate compensatory cytokine mechanisms that reduce inflammation and/or limit the biophysical consequences of interstitial TNF proteins. While the experimental preparation used by Sorkin et al. precluded long-term, sub-chronic studies of these possible dynamic interactions, the data suggest that TNF-induced ectopic activity provides the electrophysiological mechanisms for central sensitization. Thus, local release of TNF may be a key factor in the pathogenesis of neuropathic pain states following injury to peripheral nerves.

Cytokine therapy

One approach to understanding the role of cytokines in the pathogenesis of neuropathic pain would be to test the effect of selected drugs or other experimental therapies that target either the production or expression of locally-generated cytokines. The development of molecular antisense probes targeted at specific cytokine mRNAs will certainly result in improved insights into cytokine mechanisms of nociception and, hopefully, effective approaches to human therapy. To date, however, only more circumvent approaches have been published.

Thalidomide is a drug that inhibits the production of TNF in activated macrophages [58, 59] and has been shown to be useful clinically in the treatment of leprosy and graft-versus-host disease [60–64] and in painful conditions such as AIDS [65] in which TNF has been suspected to be a key pathogenic component. It was reasoned that thalidomide therapy may also reduce thermal hyperalgesia and mechanical allodynia in rats with chronic constriction injury [37]. In rats in which treatment with thalidomide was started preoperatively, there was diminished mechanical allodynia and thermal hyperalgesia during the early stage of CCI neuropathy. TNF immunohistochemistry revealed reduced cellular immunoreactivity on day 5 post-surgery as compared to sham-treated animals. The pathological vascular changes were also reduced in thalidomide-treated rats. Starting treatment with thalidomide at a time-point when hyperalgesia was already present did not alter the course of the pain-related behavior. It was concluded that preemptive treatment with a substance that blocks production of TNF reduces pain-related symptoms and pathological vascular changes in the chronic constriction injury model of neuropathic pain. Therapy started at a later time, for example after endothelial activation and the initial release of TNF by injured Schwann cells, may not be sufficient to block the cascade of cytokine events associated with the development of chronic pain.

Interleukin-10 is an endogenous anti-inflammatory peptide that down-regulates proinflammatory cytokines [66] and functionally inhibits TNF action [67]. We reasoned that if IL-10 was delivered to the focus of the peripheral nerve injury in CCI neuropathy that there would be decreased macrophage recruitment, endoneurial TNF expression, and thermal hyperalgesia [68]. To test the hypothesis, 250 ng of IL-10 (Genzyme) in a 10 µl volume was injected into rat sciatic nerve at the time of CCI surgery. Control groups received vehicle and CCI surgery or IL-10 and sham surgery. In IL-10-treated CCI animals, thermal hyperalgesia was significantly reduced at days 3, 5, and 9 following CCI relative to vehicle-injected CCI animals (Fig. 11). IL-10 injection alone without CCI surgery had no significant effect on behavioral differences when compared to the unoperated limb. Histological sections from the peripheral nerve injury site of IL-10-treated CCI animals had decreased cell profiles immunoreactive for ED-1, a marker of recruited macrophages, at both time-points studied (two and five days post-CCI). IL-10 treatment also had decreased cell profiles of the pro-inflammatory cytokine TNF at day 2, but not day 5 post-CCI. Interestingly, the attenuation of thermal hyperalgesia extended beyond the predicted half-life of the administered IL-10, into the period when the number of TNF-positive cells was not significantly different between groups.

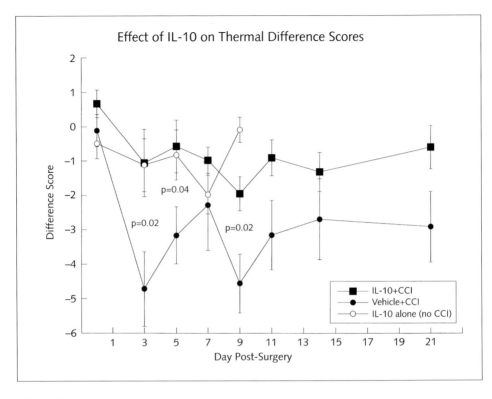

Figure 11
Thermal difference scores (experimental minus contralateral control paw latency) from rats that received CCI and injection of 10 µl of either vehicle (0.1% bovine serum albumin in 0.1M phosphate buffer) or 250 ng of IL-10. Mean ± S.E.M. difference scores throughout the experimental period. There is a significant reduction in CCI-induced hyperalgesia in the IL-10 treated animals at days 3, 4, and 9 after nerve injury.

Conclusions

The data reviewed in this chapter support the following hypotheses on the role of cytokines at the nerve injury site and their roles in the pathogenesis of neuropathic pain states. Initial production of TNF at the site of nerve injury is a critical factor in the cascade of events leading to neuropathic pain states. Local TNF influences later sequelae such as the inflammatory response raised against the injury and the development of nociceptive behaviors. It appears that TNF is a common denominator of events that have been considered important to the development of pain states. These events include the presence of edema and reduced nerve blood flow at the injury site [11] and resulting lowered oxygen levels [69], cytotoxicity of endoneurial components such as Schwann cells and some axons [43, 52], the upregulation of nerve growth factor production [70] with associated hyperalgesia actions [71], and the upregulation of intracellular adhesion molecules and macrophage chemotaxis [25]. Pharmacological interference with any link in this chain of events has potential therapeutic value.

We do not suggest that it is only through these mechanisms that neuropathic pain develops, or that Wallerian degeneration is the only pathological change correlated with painful nerve injury. However, to the extent that nerve injury triggers cellular inflammation in the environment of sensory axons, hyperalgesia will be developed during the period of axonal degeneration and may progress to neuropathic pain if reinforced by other mechanisms of signaling and chemical change in afferent sensory pathways.

References

1   Wagner R, DeLeo JA, Heckman HM, Myers RR (1995) Peripheral nerve pathology following sciatic nerve cryoneurolysis: Relationship to neuropathic behaviors. *Exp Neurol* 133: 256–264

2   Scadding JW (1994) Peripheral Neuropathies. In: PD Wall and R Melzack (eds): *Textbook of pain*. Churchill Livingston, Edinburgh, 667–683

3   Thomas PK (1979) Painful neuropathies. In: Bonica JJ (ed): *Painful neuropathies 3*. Raven Press, New York, 103–110

4   Dyck PJ, Lambert EH, O'Brien PC (1976) Pain in peripheral neuropathy related to rate and kind of fiber degeneration. *Neurology* 26: 466–471

5   Asbury AK, Fields HL (1984) Pain due to peripheral nerve damage: an hypothesis. *Neurol* 34: 1587–1590

6   Chaplan SR, Bach SW, Pogrel JW, Chung JM, Yaksh TL (1994) Quantitative assessment of tactile allodynia in the rat paw. *J Neurosci Meth* 53: 55–63

7   Hargreaves K, Dubner R, Brown F, Flores C, Joris J (1988) A new and sensitive method for measuring thermal nociception in cutaneous hyperalgesia. *Pain* 32: 77–88

8   Bennett GJ, Xie Y-K (1988) A peripheral mononeuropathy in rat that produces disorders of pain sensation like those seen in man. *Pain* 33: 498–507

9   Kim SH, Chung JM (1992) An experimental for peripheral neuropathy produced by segmental spinal nerve ligation in the rat. *Pain* 50: 355–362

10 Myers RR, Heckman HM, Powell HC (1996) Axonal viability and the persistence of thermal hyperalgesia after partial freeze lesions of nerve. *J Neurol Sci* 139: 28–38

11 Myers RR, Yamamoto T, Yaksh TL, Powell HC (1993) The role of focal nerve ischemia and Wallerian degeneration in peripheral nerve injury producing hyperesthesia. *Anesthesiology* 78: 308–316

12 Basbaum AI, Gautron M, Jazat F, Mayes M, Guilbaud G (1991) The spectrum of fiber

loss in a model of neuropathic pain in the rat: an electron microscopic study. *Pain* 47: 359–367

13 Coggeshall RE, Dougherty PM, Pover CM, Carlton SM (1993) Is large myelinated fiber loss associated with hyperalgesia in a model of experimental peripheral neuropathy in the rat? *Pain* 52: 233–242

14 Sommer C, Galbraith JA, Heckman HM, Myers RR (1993) Pathology of experimental compression neuropathy producing hyperesthesia. *J Neuropath Exp Neurol* 52: 223–233

15 Sommer C, Lalonde A, Heckman HM, Rodriguez M, Myers RR (1995) Quantitative neuropathology of a focal nerve injury causing hyperalgesia. *J Neuropath Exp Neurol* 54: 635–643

16 Yaksh TL, Yamamoto T, Myers RR (1991) Pharmacology of nerve compression evoked hyperesthesia. In: Willis W (ed): *Hyperalgesia and allodynia*. Raven Press, New York, 245–258

17 Ambron RT, Walters ET (1996) Priming events and retrograde injury signals. *Mol Neurobiol* 13: 61–79

18 Cragg BG (1970) What is the signal for chromatolysis? *Brain Res* 23: 1–21

19 Wu W, Mathew TC, Miller FD (1993) Evidence that the loss of homeostatic signals induces regeneration-associated alteration in neuronal gene expression. *Dev Biol* 158: 445–466

20 Fukuoka H, Kawatani M, Hisamitsu T, Takeshige C (1994) Cutaneous hyperalgesia induced by peripheral injection of interleukin 1β in the rat. *Brain Res* 657: 133–140

21 Woolf CJ, Allchorne A, Safieh-Garabedian B, Poole S (1997) Cytokines, nerve growth factor and inflammatory hyperalgesia: the contribution of tumor necrosis factor α. *Br J Pharmacol* 121: 417–424

22 White DM (1977) Release of substance P from peripheral sensory nerve terminals. *J Periph Nerv Sys* 2: 191–201

23 Johnson D, Krenger W (1992) Interactions of mast cells with the nervous system – recent advances. *Neurochem Res* 17: 939–951

24 Beuche W, Friede RL (1984) The role of non-resident cells in Wallerian degeneration. *J Neurocytol* 13: 767–796

25 Griffin JW, George R, Ho T (1993) Macrophage systems in peripheral nerves. A review. *J Neuropath Exp Neurol* 52: 553–560

26 Perry VH, Brown MC, Lunn ER, Gordon S (1990) Evidence that very slow Wallerian degeneration in C57BL/Ola mice is an intrinsic property of the peripheral nerve. *Eur J Neurosci* 2: 802–812

27 Brown MC, Perry VH, Lunn ER, Gordon S, Heumann R (1991) Macrophage dependence of peripheral sensory nerve regeneration: possible involvement of nerve growth factor. *Neuron* 6: 359–370

28 Lyon M, Ogunkolade B, Brown M, Atherton D, Perry V (1993) A gene affecting Wallerian nerve degeneration maps distally on mouse chromosome 4. *Proc Natl Acad Sci USA* 90: 9717–9720

29   Myers RR, Heckman HM, Rodriguez M (1996) Reduced hyperalgesia in nerve-injured WLD mice: Relationship to nerve fiber phagocytosis, axonal degeneration and regeneration in normal mice. *Exp Neurol* 141: 94–101.

30   Ramer MS, French GD, Bisby MA (1997) Wallerian degeneration is required for both neuropathic pain and sympathetic sprouting into the DRG. *Pain* 72: 71–78

31   Bisby MA, Tetzlaff W, Brown MC (1995) Cell body response to injury in motoneurons and primary sensory neurons of a mutant mouse. Ola (Wld), in which Wallerian degeneration is delayed. *J Comp Neurol* 359: 653–662

32   Bisby MA, Chen S (1990) Delayed Wallerian degeneration in sciatic nerves of C57BL/Ola mice is associated with impaired regeneration of sensory axons. *Brain Res* 530: 117–120

33   Chen S, Bisby MA (1993) Impaired motor axon regeneration in C57BL/Ola mouse. *J Comp Neurol* 333: 449–454

34   McLachlan EM, Janig W, Devor M, Michaelis M (1993) Peripheral nerve injury triggers noradrenergic sprouting within dorsal root ganglia. *Nature* 363: 543–546

35   Adams DO, Hamilton TA (1988) Phagocytic cells: Cytotoxic activities of macrophages. In: Gallen JI, Goldstein M, Snyderman R (eds): *Inflammation: Basic principles and clinical correlates*. Raven Press, New York, 471–492

36   Heumann R, Lindholm D, Bandtlow C (1987) Differential regulation of mRNA encoding nerve growth factor and its receptor in rat sciatic nerve during development, degeneration, and regeneration: role of macrophages. *Proc Natl Acad Sci USA* 84: 8735–8739

37   Sommer C, Marziniak M, Myers RR (1998) The effect of thalidomide treatment on vascular pathology and hyperalgesia caused by chronic constriction injury of rat nerve. *Pain* 14: 83–92

38   Hartung HP, Jung S, Stoll G, Zielasek J, Schmidt B, Archelos JJ, Toyka KV (1992) Inflammatory mediators in demyelinating disorders of the CNS and PNS. *J Neuroimmunol* 40: 197–210

39   Raine CS (1994) The Dale E. McFarlin Memorial Lecture: The immunology of the multiple sclerosis lesion. *Ann Neurol* 36: S61–S72

40   Merrill JE (1992) Proinflammatory and antiinflammatory cytokines in multiple sclerosis and central nervous system acquired immunodeficiency syndrome. *J Immunotherapy* 12: 167–170

41   Griffin JW, George R, Lobato C, Tyor WR, Yan LC, Glass JD (1992) Macrophage responses and myelin clearance during Wallerian degeneration: relevance to immune-mediated demyelination. *J Neuroimmunol* 40: 153–166

42   Tyor WR, Wesselingh SL, Griffin JW, McArthur JC, Griffin DE (1995) Unifying hypothesis for the pathogenesis of HIV-associated dementia complex, vacuolar myelopathy and sensory neuropathy. *J AIDS Hum Retroviral* 9: 379–388

43   Redford EJ, Hall SM, Smith KJ (1995) Vascular changes and demyelination induced by the intraneural injection of tumour necrosis factor. *Brain* 118: 869–878

44   Said G, Hontebeyrie-Joskowicz M (1992) Nerve lesions induced by macrophage activation. *Res Immunol* 143: 589–599

45   Powell HC, Myers RR (1996) The axon in Guillain-Barre syndrome: Immune target or innocent bystander? *Ann Neurol* 39: 4–5

46   Sorkin LS, Xiao W-H, Wagner R, Myers RR (1997) Tumor necrosis factor-α induces ectopic activity in nociceptive primary afferent fibers. *Neuroscience* 81: 255–262

47   Nukada H, McMorran PD (1994) Perivascular demyelination and intramyelinic oedema in reperfusion nerve injury. *J Anat* 185: 259–266

48   Eliav E, Ruda MA, Bennett GJ (1996) An experimental neuritis of the rat sciatic nerve produces ipsilateral hindpaw allodynia and hyperalgesia. *Soc Neurosci Abs* 22: 865

49   Wagner R, Myers RR (1996) Schwann cells produce tumor necrosis factor α: Expression in injured and non-injured nerves. *Neurosci* 73: 625–629.

50   Bolin LM, Verity AN, Silver JE, Shooter EM, Abrams JS (1995) Interleukin-6 production by Schwann cells and induction in sciatic nerve injury. *J Neurochem* 64: 850–858

51   Kurek JB, Austin L, Cheema SS, Bartlett PF, Murphy M (1966) Up-regulation of leukaemia inhibitory factor and interleukin-6 in transected sciatic nerve and muscle following denervation. *Neuromusc Disord* 6: 105–114

52   Wagner R, Myers RR (1996) Endoneurial injection of TNF-α produces neuropathic pain behaviors. *NeuroReport* 7: 2897–2901

53   Cunha FQ, Poole S, Lorenzetti B, Ferreira SH (1992) The pivotal role of tumor necrosis factor α in the development of inflammatory hyperalgesia. *Br J Pharmacol* 107: 660–664

54   Devor M, Govrin-Lippmann R, Angelides K (1993) Na+ channel immunolocalization in peripheral mammalian axons and changes following nerve injury and neuroma formation. *J Neurosci* 13: 1976–1992

55   Baldwin L, Stolowitz ML, Hood L, Wisnieski BJ (1996) Structural changes of tumor necrosis factor α associated with membrane insertion and channel formation. *Proc Natl Acad Sci USA* 93: 1021–1026

56   Baldwin RL, Chang MP, Bramhill J, Graves S, Bonavida B, Wisnieski BJ (1988) Capacity of tumor necrosis factor to bind and penetrate membranes is pH dependent. *J Immunol* 141: 2352–2357

57   Kagan BL, Baldwin RL, Munoz D, Wisnieski BJ (1992) Formation of ion-permeable channels by tumor necrosis factor-α. *Science* 255: 1427–1430

58   Sampaio EP, Sarno EN, Gililly RA, Cohn Z, Kaplan G (1991) Thalidomide selectively inhibits tumor necrosis factor α production by stimulated human monocytes. *J Exp Med* 173: 699–703

59   Barnes PF, Chatterjee D, Brennan PJ, Rea TH, Modlin RL (1992) Tumor necrosis factor production in patients with leprosy. *Infect Immunol* 60: 1441–1446

60   Kaplan G (1993) Recent advances in cytokine therapy in leprosy. *J Infect Dis* 167: S18–S22

61   Sampaio EP, Kaplan G, Miranda A, Nery JA, Miguel CP, Viana SM, Sarno EN (1993) The influence of thalidomide on the clinical and immunologic manifestation of erythema nodosum leprosum. *J Infect Dis* 168: 408–414

62 Heney D, Norfolk D, Wheeldon J, Bailey C, Lewis I, Barnard D (1991) Thalidomide treatment for chronic graft-versus-host disease. *Br J Haematol* 78: 23–27

63 Vogelsang GB, Hess AD, Friedman KJ, Santos GW (1989) Therapy of chronic graft-vs-host disease in a rat model. *Blood* 74: 507–511

64 Parker PM, Chao N, Nademanee A O'Donnell MR, Schmide GM, Snyder DS, Stein AS Smith EP, Molina A, Stepan DE et al (1995) Thalidomide as salvage therapy for chronic graft-versus-host disease. *Blood* 86: 3604–3609

65 Georghiou PR and Alworth AM (1992) Thalidomide in painful AIDS-associated proctitis. *J Infect Dis* 166: 939–940

66 Fiorentino DF, Zlotnik A, Mosmann TR, Howard M, O'Garra A (1991) IL-10 inhibits cytokine production by activated macrophages. *J Immunol* 147: 3815–3822

67 Poole S, Cunha FQ, Selkirk S, Lorenzetti BB, Ferreira SH (1995) Cytokine-mediated inflammatory hyperalgesia limited by interleukin-10. *Brit J Pharm* 115: 684–688

68 Wagner R, Janjigian M, Myers RR (1998) Anti-inflammatory Interleukin-10 therapy in CCI neuropathy decreases thermal hyperalgesia, macrophage recruitment, and endoneurial TNF-α expression. *Pain* 14: 35–42

69 Ertel W, Morrison MH, Ayala A, Chaudry IH (1995) Hypoxemia in the absence of blood loss or significant hypotension causes inflammatory cytokine release. *Am J Physiol* 269: R160–R166

70 Hattori A, Hayashi K, Kohno M (1996) Tumor necrosis factor (TNF) stimulates the production of nerve growth factor in fibroblasts via the 55kDa type 1 TNF receptor. *FEBS Letters* 379: 157–160

71 Rueff A, Dawaon AJLR, Mendell LM (1996) Characteristics of nerve growth factor induced hyperalgesia in adult rats: dependence on enhanced bradykinin-1 receptor activity but not neurokinin-1 receptor activation. *Pain* 66: 359–372

Proinflammatory cytokines and glial cells: Their role in neuropathic pain

Joyce A. DeLeo and Raymond W. Colburn

Dartmouth-Hitchcock Medical Center, Departments of Anesthesiology and Pharmacology, 1 Medical Center Drive, HB 7125, Lebanon, NH, 03756, USA

Introduction

Neuropathic pain, or chronic pain due to nerve injury, is a prevalent condition for which currently there is no effective treatment. These neuropathic pain syndromes include deafferentation pain, diabetic, cancer and ischemic neuropathies, phantom limb pain, trigeminal neuralgia, postherpetic neuralgias and nerve injury caused by surgery or trauma [1]. Neuropathic pain is not only chronic and intractable, it is debilitating and causes extreme physical, psychological and social distress. In an effort to provide even temporary relief, narcotics (opioids) are often used inappropriately and in excess. Even if opioids provide some initial relief, tolerance and physical dependence are major limitations to their continued use. Clearly, development of non-opioid and non-addictive treatments for neuropathic pain would offer tremendous benefit to chronic pain patients. Our laboratory has focused on understanding mechanisms that lead to neuropathic pain. This knowledge may then translate into development of new, effective approaches for treatment and even prevention of chronic pain syndromes.

To investigate mechanisms of neuropathic pain, our laboratory developed and characterized reliable neuropathy models termed sciatic cryoneurolysis (SCN) [2–4] and spinal nerve cryoneurolysis (SPCN) [5, 6] in the rat. The models produce a focal nerve lesion by exposure and freezing of the sciatic nerve (SCN) or the more proximal L5 spinal nerve (SPCN). The models have proved ideal for the study of neuropathic pain due to the creation of predictable and robust pain behaviors. Using these neurolysis models, the chronic constriction [7] and the spinal nerve tight ligation models [8] we found evidence that immune cell activation and immune cell products (cytokines) may contribute to generation of chronic pain states. When we combine our data with reports from investigators using acute pain models [9], we have evidence for a central, spinal role of cytokines in the etiology of chronic pain states.

Cytokines

Cytokines, which act on many different cell types, are involved in immunity and inflammation where they regulate the amplitude and duration of a response. Our laboratory has recently focused on the role of proinflammatory cytokines: Interleukin (IL)-1, IL-6, and tumor necrosis factor-α (TNF-α) in the development of chronic neuropathic pain.

Interleukin-1

IL-1 has multiple roles in inflammation and in the immune response. Of the two forms of IL-1, IL-1α and IL-1β, IL-1β is the predominate molecule in brain tissue [10]. IL-1β is synthesized not only by peripheral immune cells, but also by activated astrocytes and microglial cells [11, 12] and neurons [13, 14]. IL-1β has immunogenic activity, causing release of prostaglandins, IL-6, and IL-8 from monocytes and endothelial cells. IL-1 mediates its activities through receptors (R) on the cell membrane, either IL-1R type I (IL-1α) or type II (IL-1β) [15].

With regard to neuropathic pain, we know that IL-1β production is enhanced in the periphery following crush injury to a peripheral nerve and in microglia and astrocytes after CNS trauma [16]. IL-1β mimics the hyperalgesic action of illness-inducing substances (lithium chloride and endotoxin) which adds particular significance to the role of cytokines in nociception. IL-1 hyperalgesia is abolished by the systemic administration of an IL-1 receptor antagonist (IL-1ra) [17]. Oka et al. have demonstrated that intracerebroventricular injection of IL-1β induces hyperalgesia and enhances nociceptive neuronal responses of trigeminal nucleus caudalis in rats [18, 19]. Conversely, when recombinant human IL-1β (rhIL-1β) is microinjected specifically into the ventromedial hypothalamus, analgesia was produced [20]. Relevant to nociceptive processing, IL-1β facilitates afferent sensory transmission in the somatosensory cortex [21]. It is also likely that certain cytokines, like IL-1β, are involved in synaptic plasticity and hyperexcitability due to their dose-dependent capacity to produce long-term potentiation in slice preparations, that pathophysiologically correlates to spinal sensitization [10, 22].

Interleukin-6

IL-6, along with IL-1 and TNF, is one of the mediators of the acute phase response of inflammation. In addition to its role in the acute inflammatory response, it plays an important part in host defense and chronic immune responses. Over-expression of IL-6 is implicated in diseases such as systemic lupus erythematosus and rheumatoid arthritis [15]. IL-6 exerts its activity through binding to a high affinity receptor complex comprising an 80 kDa receptor protein (IL-6R) and 130 kDa signal trans-ducing glycoprotein (gp-130) [23]. IL-6 is synthesized by mononuclear phagocytes, vascular endothelial cells, fibroblasts and other cells in response to IL-1 and TNF [28].

Following axotomy or a freeze lesion of a spinal nerve, an increase in IL-6 mRNA is one of the earliest changes observed in the spinal cord and dorsal root ganglia [24, 25]. In addition, IL-6 message is induced in Schwann cells distal to a crush injury [26]. *In vitro*, IL-6 is produced by cultured astrocytes and microglia [27, 28]. In vivo, IL-6 may act as an early activating signal for glial cells. It has been shown that IL-6 expression in transgenic mice causes reactive astrocytes and an increase in microglial cells [29]. This is of interest since we have observed a robust glial activation of both astrocytes and microglia following a nerve injury that caus-es neuropathic pain behaviors in rats [6, 30].

Increasing evidence supports a role for cytokines as chemical signals/ neuro-modulators in the central nervous system (CNS) in normal and under pathological conditions. Intracerebroventricular [31] and intrathecal [32] administration of IL-6 induces thermal hyperalgesia and mechanical allodynia in normal rats. These data support a role of IL-6 in direct nociceptive processing. It has also been demonstrat-ed that IL-6 significantly enhances the response to N-methyl-D-aspartate (NMDA) in cultured rat cerebellar granule neurons [33]. This finding has important func-tional implications under conditions of elevated IL-6 protein which we have observed following nerve injury. Past research of chronic pain mechanisms has focused on the involvement of glutamate, acting mainly via the NMDA receptor. Researchers have shown that antagonists of the glutamate NMDA receptor mitigate pain behaviors in animal models of neuropathic pain [34, 35]. Some of the less selec-tive NMDA receptor antagonists are currently in clinical trials for treatment of chronic neuropathic pain [36].

Tumor necrosis factor-α

The tumor necrosis factors include TNFα (or cachectin) and TNFβ (or lymphotox-in) [37, 38]. In common with all cytokines, interaction with a specific receptor is necessary for a biological response. Its potency is such that occupancy of as little as 5% of its receptors produces a biological response [39]. There are two distinct cell-surface receptors, p55 and p75 [40, 41]. Soluble, truncated versions of membrane TNF receptors are elevated in many autoimmune and inflammatory conditions and are thought to be involved in regulating TNF activity [42, 43]. These tumor necro-sis factors produce a variety of similar, but not identical, biological effects. These factors are "proinflammatory cytokines" since they have a role in initiating (along with IL-1) the cascade of other cytokines and growth factors that participate in the immune inflammatory response.

Like IL-1, TNFα is implicated in enhanced pain responses following administration of illness-inducing substances [17]. When a TNFα antagonist, TNF-binding protein (TNF-bp), is administered systemically, the hyperalgesia observed after lipopolysaccharide (LPS, a bacterial cell wall component) is completely eliminated, suggesting that TNF, like IL-1, is a critical cytokine for the induction of LPS-induced hyperalgesia. In addition, treatment of rheumatoid arthritis with a recombinant human TNF receptor (p75)-Fc fusion protein significantly improves inflammatory symptoms [44].

Studies have revealed that cytokines may affect neuronal excitability either directly or indirectly via an alteration of neuron-glia interaction. TNFα induces an increase in intracellular calcium and a depolarization in astrocytes with the consequence of disturbing voltage-dependent glial function such as local ion concentrations and glutamate uptake [45]. The neurotoxic effects of TNFα may be due in part to its ability to inhibit glutamate uptake by astrocytes, which in turn may result in excitotoxic concentrations of glutamate in synapses [46]. This glutamate enhancing action may also be of importance in chronic pain following nerve injury. Similarly, TNFα induces substance P, a major pain mediator, in sympathetic ganglia [47].

Spinal cytokine characterization in neuropathic pain models

The classic example of scientific identification of a new pathophysiological network is to first identify and characterize previously unmeasured components in an accepted animal model of the disease process in question. Using immunohistochemistry, we characterized the expression of a variety of cytokines and growth factors in the spinal cord following different nerve lesions that produce neuropathic pain-like behaviors. Of interest to the focus of this chapter, we reported incremental increases in spinal IL-6-like immunoreactivity (LI) expression following sciatic cryoneurolysis which closely correlated with the onset and duration of mechanical allodynia [32] (Fig. 1). Subsequent to this study, we extended our investigation to include spinal IL-1β and TNFα expression in both the sciatic cryoneurolysis and chronic constriction injury models [48]. We observed minimal, diffuse cytokine LI in lumbar spinal tissue from normal, unlesioned rats. In contrast, using cell profile quantification we demonstrated increases in lumbar spinal IL-1β and TNFα LI in both mononeuropathy models studied (Figs. 2, 3 and Tab. 1, 2).

These immunohistochemical data provide evidence that specific cytokines are elevated in the spinal cord following peripheral nerve lesions that reliably result in neuropathic behaviors. However, one of the challenges in cytokine research which has hampered major advances in the localization of these proteins in the central nervous system is the absence of purified and standardized cytokine antibodies. This is particularly relevant when utilizing immunohistochemistry and enzyme-linked immunosorbent assay (ELISA) as detection methods for cytokines. The rate of false

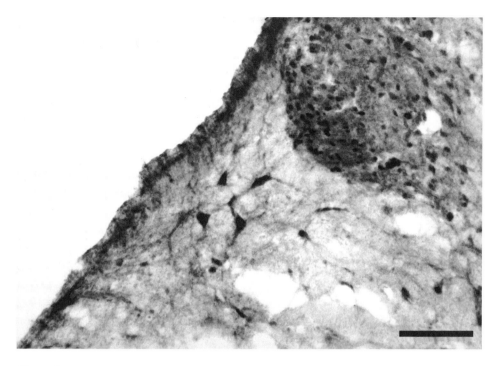

Figure 1
Representative IL-6 immunoreactivity in the dorsal horn of the spinal cord three days after sciatic cryoneurolysis (bar = 20 microns).

positives is high especially when using ELISA methodology since it is difficult to distinguish true positivity in a colormetric technique without the benefit of morphological visualization. Suppliers of antibodies incorporate varied standards for purification and quality control of their products. We have embarked on an ambitious project where we are comparing seven different commercial sources of proinflammatory cytokine antibodies in two models of nerve injury and in a rat model of focal CNS immune-mediated inflammation, experimental allergic encephalomyelitis (EAE), with and without preabsorbing with the specific rat immunogen. At the study's end, a standard of optimum staining for each cytokine antibody will be obtained that can be utilized by other investigators performing CNS cytokine immunohistochemistry and ELISAs. As the cytokine field continues to expand, we can use the identical system for future analysis of new antibodies as they become available.

The next phase in our quest to understand the neuroimmunological events that occur in response to nerve injury is to determine the cellular mechanisms responsible for increases in spinal cytokines.

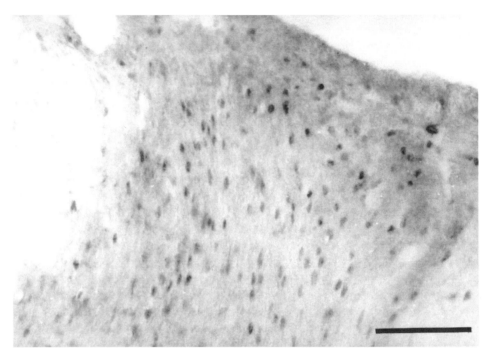

Figure 2
Representative photomicrograph of ipsilateral dorsal horn IL-1β-like immunoreactivity three
days after sciatic cryoneurolysis (bar = 20 microns).
Reproduced with permission [48].

Table 1 - Average cell profiles containing punctate IL-1β staining[1]

Group (N ≥ 3)	Ipsilateral dorsal horn	Contralateral dorsal horn	Ipsilateral ventral horn	Contralateral ventral horn
Normal	0.15 (0.17)	0.00 (0)	0.13 (0.08)	0.00 (0)
CCI	36.00** (4.2)	22.67* (6.12)	15.00 (6.12)	15.00* (4.6)
3-day post-SCN	50.45** (8.7)	32.58** (8.5)	5.48* (1.1)	3.62* (0.53)
14-day post-SCN	40.44* (11.0)	36.33* (9.02)	1.56 (0.68)	1.22 (0.68)
35-day post-SCN	76.60** (15.7)	53.94** (6.9)	3.71 (1.1)	2.27 (0.43)

[1]Average of three lumbar sections/animal (± SEM)
*$p < 0.05$ using multiple regression with normal group as reference category
**$p < 0.001$ using multiple regression with normal group as reference category.
Reproduced with permission [48].

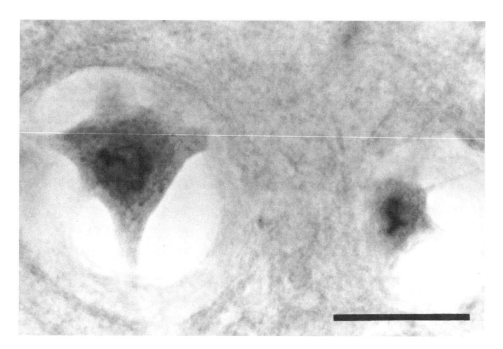

Figure 3
Representative photomicrograph of ventral horn motorneurons containing dark punctate nuclear TNFα like-immunoreactivity 14 days following sciatic cryoneurolysis (bar = 20 microns).
Reproduced with permission [48].

Table 2 - Average cell profiles containing punctate TNFα staining[1]

Group (N = 3)	Ipsilateral dorsal horn	Contralateral dorsal horn	Ipsilateral ventral horn	Contralateral ventral horn
Normal	6.00 (1.7)	2.44 (1.7)	0.00 (0)	0.00 (0)
CCI	22.00* (4.9)	12.33* (4.4)	4.89 (4.3)	2.89 (8.48)
3-day post-SCN	67.11** (13.5)	48.33** (7.6)	16.44* (4.9)	11.78* (5.7)
14-day post-SCN	122.67** (5.6)	118.89** (6.4)	16.00** (0.71)	14.22* (0.76)
35-day post-SCN	42.00* (11.0)	57.67** (4.9)	1.56 (0.4)	0.89 (0.06)

[1]*Average of three lumbar sections/animal (± SEM)*
$p < 0.05$ using multiple regression with normal group as reference category
$p < 0.001$ using multiple regression with normal group as reference category.
Reproduced with permission [Brain Research 759 (1997) 50–57].

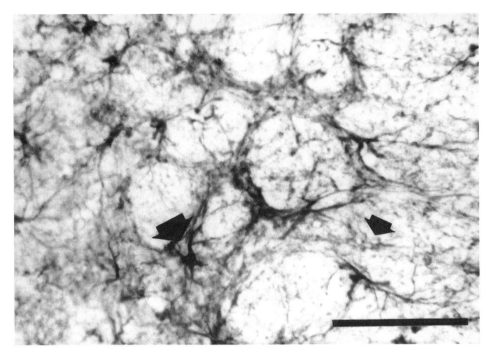

Figure 4
Double immunohistochemical labeling of cytokine expression and glial staining after spinal nerve cryoneurolysis. Astrocytic (GFAP) staining is shown in gray (small arrow), original depicted as a brown chromagen. TNFα staining is shown in black (large arrow), original depicted as a blue chromagen (bar = 20 microns).

Cellular origin of spinal cytokine expression

Double staining of cytokines and glia

In order to determine whether neurons or glia are expressing cytokines following peripheral nerve injury, we performed immunohistochemical double staining for each cytokine/growth factor and for cellular markers of astrocytes or microglia. The combinations performed were: antibodies for IL-6, IL-1, and TNFα co-localized on the same section with either anti-GFAP (glial fibrillary acidic protein) for astrocytes or anti-OX-42 for microglia using two different colored detection chromagens. Most combinations resulted in a distinct staining pattern with cytokines localized only to what appeared to be neuronal cells without detectable co-labeling with glial cells. Of particular interest, the only co-localization observed was with TNFα and GFAP (Fig. 4). TNFα staining was localized to both neurons and astrocytes but not microglia.

Table 3 - Average cell profiles containing IL-6 mRNA staining[1]

Group (N ≥ 3)	Ipsilateral dorsal horn	Contralateral dorsal horn	Ipsilateral ventral horn	Contralateral ventral horn
Normal	6.11	6.67	1.00	1.11
CCI	22.00* (4.9)	12.33* (4.4)	4.89 (4.3)	2.89 (8.48)
1-day post-SPCN	10.44	4.89	6.56	0.67
3-day post-SPCN	17.67	8.89	10.56***	2.56
10-day post-SPCN	41.11*	25.33*	9.11**	5.67**

[1]Average of three lumbar sections/animal (± SEM)
*p = 0.001, **p = 0.05, ***p = 0.05.02

Cytokine mRNA *in situ* hybridization (ISH)

To definitively determine whether cytokines are actually being produced within the CNS in response to a peripheral nerve injury, it is necessary to perform ISH. An oligonucleotide cocktail of four exons (30bp each) of IL-6 mRNA was hybridized to spinal cord tissue. Using this technique without polymerase chain reaction (PCR) amplification, we demonstrated an increase in IL-6 mRNA in the spinal cord 1, 3 and 10 days following SPCN as compared with normal rats (see Tab. 3 and Fig. 5). These data support our hypothesis that cells in the central nervous system are producing cytokines in response to a peripheral nerve injury. The next logical step is to determine what cell type (e.g. astrocyte, microglia, neuron) is producing IL-6 mRNA by performing both ISH for mRNA and immunocytochemistry on the same section using cell specific markers.

Role of glial cells in increased spinal cytokine expression

Glial cells (microglia, astrocytes, and oligodendrocytes) constitute over 70% of the total cell population in the brain and spinal cord. Once thought of as merely a physical support system for neurons, glial cells have recently come under intense scrutiny as key neuromodulatory, neurotrophic and neuroimmune elements in the CNS. Microglia, cells of monocytic origin, are the macrophages of the brain and, as such, perform a vast number of immune-related duties [49]. They form a regularly-spaced network of resident glial cells throughout the CNS. Microglia are the first cell type to respond to several types of CNS injury. Pathological stimuli provoke a graded transformation of microglia from a highly ramified resting surveillance state ulti-

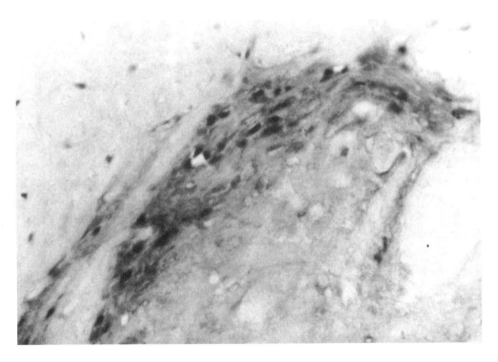

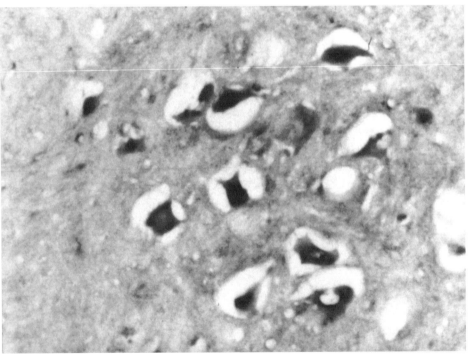

mately to a phagocytic macrophage [50]. Microglial activation involves a stereo-typic pattern of cellular responses, such as proliferation, increased expression of immunomolecules, recruitment to the site of injury, and functional changes includ-ing the release of cytotoxic and/or inflammatory mediators. During autoimmune inflammation of the nervous system, microglia both release and respond to several cytokines including IL-1, IL-6, TNFα, and interferon-γ, all of which are also instru-mental in astrocyte activation, induction of cell adhesion molecule expression and recruitment of T cell lymphocytes into the lesion [50]. In addition to the synthesis of inflammatory cytokines, microglia act as cytotoxic effector cells by releasing harmful substances including proteases, reactive oxygen intermediates, and nitric oxide (NO) [50].

Glial cells may have a role in nociceptive processing and in the thermal and mechanical hyperalgesia produced by peripheral nerve injury [51]. Glial changes in response to injury include proliferation and hypertrophy of astrocytic and microglia cells and over-expression of GFAP. GFAP increases in the spinal cord following dif-ferent nerve injuries such as CCI [52], nerve crush and axotomy [53, 54]. Follow-ing a peripheral nerve freeze lesion, immunoreactive GFAP expression increases at 14 days with a second major increase at 42 days consistent with peaks in autotomy behavior (attack of affected hind paw) and mechanical allodynia, respectively [30]. Since glial cells produce cytokines that appear to have a role in sensitization of the spinal cord, which, in turn, may initiate or sustain chronic pain it is important to determine their contribution to neuropathic pain following nerve injury.

It has been demonstrated that the neurotransmitter norepinephrine (NE) induces astrocytes to produce IL-6 [55]. This effect is dose-dependent and can be blocked by adrenergic receptor antagonists. These data have relevant implications to human neuropathic pain since one component is the phenomenon of sympathetically-main-tained pain. Sympathetic exacerbation of neuropathic pain appears to result from at least two related pathological changes: increased sympathetic input by the invasion of sympathetic fibers into the dorsal root ganglion and the up-regulation of adren-ergic receptors on afferent fibers and cell bodies [56–59]. In addition, astrocytes express receptors for NE [60], NE induces astrocyte nerve growth factor synthesis [61] and NE inhibits astrocyte expression of major histocompatibility complex (MHC) class II antigens [62]. Of interest to the differential role of glia, rat microglia do not secrete IL-6 in response to NE, TNFα or IL-1β, indicating that rat astrocytes and microglia produce IL-6 in response to different inducing stimuli [55].

Figure 5
In situ *hybridization of IL-6 mRNA expression ten days after spinal nerve cryoneurolysis in* *dorsal horn (top photo) and ventral motorneurons (bottom photo).*

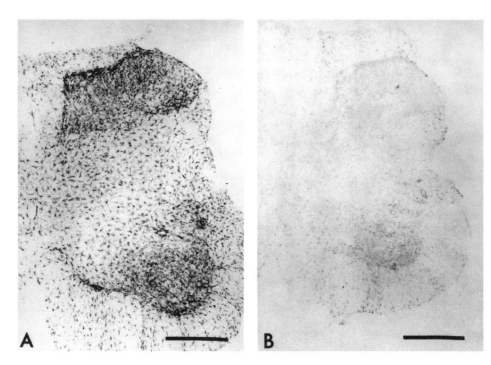

Figure 6
Ipsilateral spinal cord OX-42 ir at ten days following either SPCN with prophylactic per-
ineural saline (A) or bupivacaine (B) treatment. Note the intensity of microglial reaction in
the SPCN/saline treated animal and the relative lack of staining in the SPCN/bupivacaine
treated rat (bar = 0.5 mm). For further explanations see text.
Reproduced with permission [5].

Immunocytochemical glial characterization following nerve injury

We assessed spinal glial activation and cytokine expression following L5 spinal
nerve cryoneurolysis (SPCN) and chronic constriction injury (CCI) using immunocytochemical detection of OX-42 monoclonal antibody (microglial activation), and
glial fibrillary acidic protein antibody (GFAP; astrocytic activation) [5, 6]. Profound
microglial responses were observed ipsilaterally in the dorsal and ventral horns in
rats following SPCN (Figs. 6A and 7A). In contrast, spinal OX-42 immunoreactivity was not markedly elevated in those rats that underwent the CCI lesion five days
prior and appeared qualitatively similar to control or sham rats. In addition, neuropathic pain behaviors preceded and did not strictly correlate with microglial activation. Pain behaviors were seen to exist in the absence of microglial activation and

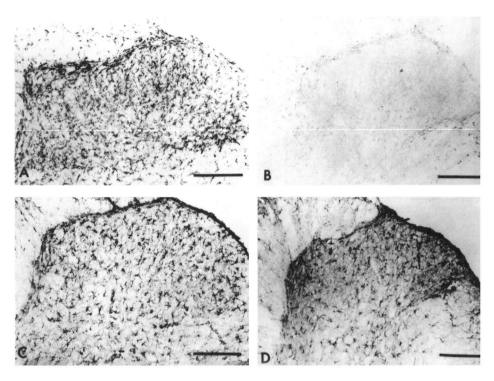

Figure 7
A–B: Ipsilateral spinal dorsal horn OX-42 ir at ten days following either SPCN with prophy-
lactic perineural saline (A), bupivacaine (B) treatments. Note the intensity of microglial reac-
tion in the SPCN/saline treated animal and the relative lack of staining in the SPCN/bupi-
vacaine treated rat.
C–D: Ipsilateral spinal dorsal horn GFAP ir in the same rats as in A–B above at ten days fol-
lowing either SPCN with prophylactic perineural saline (C), bupivacaine (D) treatments.
Note the intensity of astrocytic reaction in all treatment groups (bar = 20 microns). For fur-
ther explanations see text.
Reproduced with permission [5].

conversely, profound microglial activation was occasionally associated with a lack of pain behaviors.

A progession of astrocytic response was observed following SPCN. Little enhancement of GFAP immunoreactivity was seen at one day post sham or SPCN relative to normal animals. By ten days, there was a pronounced increase in activated astrocytes post-SPCN. GFAP expression was increased in the dorsal horn substantia gelatinosa and in the white matter immediately lateral to the dorsal horn in the CCI lesioned group (Fig. 7).

Pre-emptive bupivacaine treatment

In a second series of animals, perineural application of the amide local anesthetic, bupivacaine (1.5 mg total dose), 5 min prior to and immediately following the SPCN lesion, prevented or markedly reduced spinal microglial responses (at ten days) as compared to saline treated control animals (Figs. 6 and 7). No diminution of pain behaviors was observed in these bupivacaine treated animals despite the apparent lack of microglial activation [5]. Therefore, a causal association between microglia (using anti-OX-42 to illuminate microglial morphological responses), and the etiology of pain behaviors appears unlikely since: (1) there was no direct correlation between degree of microglial activation and severity of pain behaviors after SPCN, (2) pretreatment of the SPCN injury site with bupivacaine prevented microglial responses but did not affect the resultant pain behaviors, and (3) the CCI lesion that resulted in significant pain behaviors did not produce substantial microglial activation in the spinal cord at the time period of tissue harvest.

In addition, the observation that bupivacaine diminished spinal OX-42 expression but did not alter enhanced cytokine-like immunoreactivity following SPCN suggests that microglia are not producing proinflammatory cytokines in this *in vivo* situation; or alternatively, ramified microglia may still be producing cytokines in this scenario but the upregulation of the surface antigen CD11b (to which OX-42 binds) is downstream from this phenomenon. Thus, microglial responses may be a result of, rather than the source of, pathophysiological changes producing neuropathic pain.

Unlike the diminution of microglial activation observed following perineural bupivacaine administration, astrocytic responses were not markedly altered by this treatment (Fig. 5). These data, together with the finding that GFAP was elevated in the CCI lesioned rats, supports a role for astrocytes in neuropathic pain-related behaviors following nerve injury.

Ongoing experimental directions

To further define the signals responsible for glial activation responses and enhanced spinal cytokine expression, we are currently investigating the role of the site of lesion (distal or proximal to the dorsal root ganglion (DRG)) and the type of the nerve lesion (freeze, ligation or chemical) on spinal cytokine and glial profiles and pain-related behaviors. Our results suggest that DRG-induced production of neuroactive substances is not a critical factor in early pain behaviors, since complete dorsal root lesion produced rapid and profound pain behaviors [6]. These preliminary studies appear to further divest microglial activation responses from direct culpability in the generation neuropathic pain behaviors since dorsal root lesions were associated with minimal microglial responses while simultaneously producing robust mechanical allodynia. It is interesting to speculate as to the role of the afferent neuronal cell body (DRG) in potentiating microglial activation. Analogous to the dorsal root lesion situation, when DRG stimulatory electrical/inflammatory signals were blocked by perineural bupivacaine treatment at the time of nerve injury, spinal microglial activation was mitigated despite the presence of robust mechanical allodynia (see above). Conversely, astrocytic activation responses following dorsal root lesions were robust and similar to those seen following the same lesions at more peripheral sites with or without bupivacaine treatment.

In considering the likely underlying signals for spinal glial activation and cytokine expression following peripheral nerve injury the obvious categories include (a) disruption or exaggeration of normal axonal electrical activity, (b) disruption or augmentation of axonally transported factors, and (c) local inflammatory responses which modify (a) and (b). Ongoing signals from the periphery, both electrical and transported, may be required to maintain spinal glia in a "resting" state. For example, disruption of normal electrical activity or interruption of the axonal transport of neurotrophic factors from the periphery may lead to central neuronal changes which are readily detected by adjacent glial cells [63]. Conversely, an injury may induce exaggerated electrical signals either directly as an afferent barrage or secondary to local inflammatory neuronal sensitization [64]. A deluge of ectopic firing is likely to lead to central facilitation subsequent to primary afferent enhanced excitatory amino acid and neuropeptide release. Similarly, retrograde transport of inflammatory mediators such as activated cytokines and their receptor complexes may provoke DRG sensitization.

Astrocytes are uniquely situated to influence both neuronal excitability through synaptic glutamate handling and to direct cytokine/chemokine-induced monocyte (microglial) migration either locally or through perivascular recruitment [65–67]. Figure 8 depicts a scheme of possible glia/cytokine/glutamate interactions involved in the mechanisms of neuropathic pain. It remains unclear whether the profound ipsilateral increase in microglial cell density following various spinal nerve injuries results from significant infiltration of monocytes or from proliferation and migration of resident parenchymal microglia. Ongoing studies in our laboratory using proliferating cell markers as well as adhesion molecule antagonists will determine the relative contribution of parenchymal versus recruited monocytes involved in various nerve lesion scenarios.

The concept of experimentally interfering with astrocytic activation is attractive given our consistent finding that astrocytic responses closely correlate with cytokine expression and pain behaviors. The glutamate antagonist MK-801 has been used to mitigate astroglial GFAP expression in response to nerve injury; however, spinal cytokine levels and pain behaviors were not monitored in that study [68]. General metabolic glial inhibitors have been used to examine the possible role of glia in pain processing [51, 69]. These studies provide encouraging evidence for astrocytic involvement in pain processing possibly via cytokines and NO interactions. How-

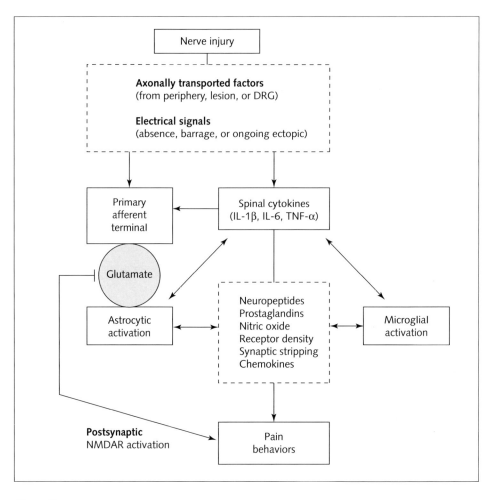

Figure 8
Schematic diagram of possible glia/cytokine/glutamate interactions in neuropathic pain.
(DRG, Dorsal root ganglion; NMDAR, N-methyl-D-aspartate receptor)

ever, direct quantitative and morphological evidence for selective and specific astrocytic inhibition remains to be put forward.

Role of cytokines in the generation of chronic pain

We hypothesize that proinflammatory cytokines have a pain facilitory effect following nerve injury by activating peripheral and central neurotransmission. Proinflammatory cytokines can cause direct sensitization of peripheral nerves. It has been demonstrated that TNFα when applied on the sciatic nerve, evokes spontaneous firing of nociceptive primary afferent fibers in a dose-dependent manner [70]. In addition, mechanical threshold to a non-noxious stimulus is decreased following intradermal injection of TNFα [70, 71].

In addition to a direct sensitizing peripheral effect, proinflammatory cytokine production and expression is enhanced centrally in response to a peripheral nerve injury. The mechanisms and signals responsible for this phenomenon are currently unknown. However, central biochemical changes in other neurotransmitter systems following nerve injury have been known for some time [72–74]. As previously mentioned, it is likely that certain cytokines are involved in synaptic plasticity and hyperexcitability which can lead to spinal sensitization. Additionally, cytokines may be early activators in a pathological cascade of events following nerve injury. Cytokine activation may indirectly induce the expression of final common mediators in pain transmission, such as glutamate and nitric oxide. Lewin and Mendell have postulated that nerve injury gives rise to inflammation and release of inflammatory mediators, i.e. cytokines, which cause the release of nerve growth factor in the periphery (NGF). NGF then induces an increase in spinal sensitizing neuropeptides like substance P and calcitonin gene-related peptide (CGRP). They have demonstrated that NGF-induced thermal hyperalgesia is mediated by glutamate NMDA receptors [75]. There is also evidence that IL-1β interacts with the NMDA receptor since it has been shown that IL-1β attenuates glutamate-induced neurodegeneration [76]. A scheme is depicted in Figure 9 of possible mechanisms of cytokine-dependent sensory consequences following nerve injury that may involve the periphery, DRG (cell body) and spinal cord.

Conclusions

Consideration of proinflammatory cytokines produced by immune cells in the CNS or periphery as mediators of pain facilitation has clinical significance. Insight gained from animal pain models could be exploited to develop novel inhibitors of immune cell activation to be used either directly or in a "cocktail" combined with more traditional interventional methods for the treatment or prevention of chronic pain. A novel pharmacological approach has been proposed using specific cytokine-suppressive anti-inflammatory drugs (CSAIDs). Proinflammatory cytokine production is regulated at the transcriptional and translational level and specific agents are now being discovered which inhibit their production.

The finding that there exists functional and biochemical changes that involve the immune system in animal models of chronic pain probably is applicable to human pain syndromes. As these neuroimmune mechanisms involved in the establishment of chronic pain become more apparent, new targets for drug delivery may

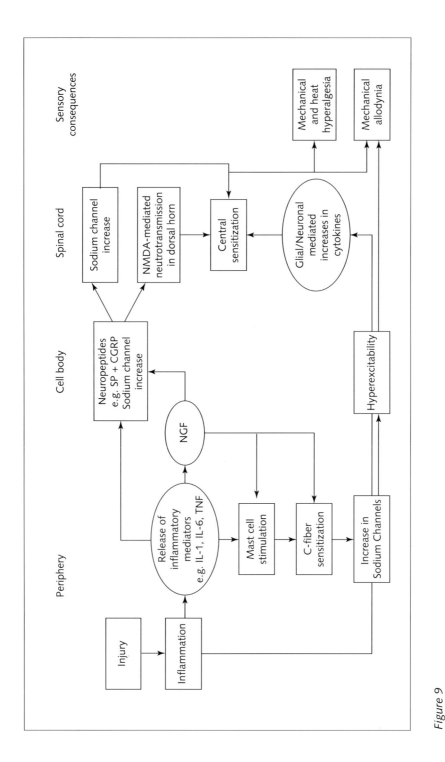

Figure 9

Schematic diagram of possible mechanisms of cytokine-dependent sensory consequences following nerve injury.
(NGF, Nerve growth factor; SP, Substance P; CGRP, Calcitonin gene-related peptide; NMDA, N-methyl-D-aspartate).
Adapted from [77].

be realized. These agents may act beyond the conventional receptor, enzyme, or channel and may modify adaptive changes in nociceptive circuits that underlie chronic pain.

Acknowledgements
The authors would like to thank Amy Rickman for technical assistance, Lisa Wirth for editorial assistance, Dr. William F. Hickey for antibodies and glial expertise; Dr. Mark E. Splaine for statistical consultation; and the following for grant support: National Institute of Drug Abuse grants DA10042 and DA11276 (JAD) and DA05731-F31 (RWC) and the National Institute of Arthritis and Musculoskeletal and Skin Diseases (JAD: AR44757) and the Orthopaedic Research and Education Foundation (JAD).

References

1   Loeser JD. (1990) Peripheral nerve disorders (peripheral neuropathies). In: Bonica J (ed): The management of pain,. 2nd ed. Lea and Febiger, Pennsylvania, 211–219

2   DeLeo JA, Coombs DW (1991) Autotomy and decreased substance P following peripheral cryogenic nerve lesion. *Cryobiol* 28: 460–466

3   DeLeo JA, Coombs DW, Willenbring SW, Colburn RW, Fromm C, Wagner R, Twitchell BB (1994) Characterization of a neuropathic pain model: Sciatic cryoneurolysis in the rat. *Pain* 56: 9–16.

4   Willenbring S, DeLeo JA, Coombs DW (1994) Differential behavioral outcomes in the sciatic cryoneurolysis model of neuropathic pain in rats. *Pain* 58: 135–140

5   Colburn RW, DeLeo JA, Rickman AJ, Yeager MP, Kwon P, Hickey WF (1997) Dissociation of microglial activation and neuropathic pain behaviors following peripheral nerve injury in the rat. *J Neuroimmunol* 79: 163–175

6   Colburn RW, DeLeo JA, Rickman AJ (1997) The effect of site vs. type of nerve injury on glial activation, spinal cytokine expression and behavior in the rat. *Soc for Neurosci Abstr*, New Orleans, LA

7   Bennett GJ, Xie YK (1988) A peripheral mononeuropathy in rat that produces disorders of pain sensation like those seen in man. *Pain* 33: 87–107

8   Kim SH, Chung JM (1992) An experimental model for peripheral neuropathy produced by segmental spinal nerve ligation in the rat. *Pain* 50: 355–363

9   Woolf CJ, Allchorne A, Safieh-Garabedian B, Poole S (1997) Cytokines, nerve growth factor and inflammatory hyperalgesia: the contribution of tumour necrosis factor-α. *Brit J Pharm* 121: 417–424

10   Rothwell NJ (1991) Functions and mechanisms of interleukin-1 in the brain. *Trends Pharmacol Sci* 12: 430–436

11   Fontana A, Kristensen F, Dubs R, Gemsa D, Weber E (1992) Production of

prostaglandin E and an interleukin-1 like factor by cultured astrocytes and C_6 glioma cells. *J Immunol* 129: 2413–2419

12 Giulian D, Baker TJ, Shih L-CN, Lachman LB (1986) Interleukin-1 of the central nervous system is produced by ameboid microglia. *J Exp Med* 164: 594–604

13 Farrar WL, Hill JM, Harel-Bellan A, Vinocour M (1987) The immunological brain. *Immunol Rev* 100: 361–378

14 Lechan RM, Toni R, Clark BD, Cannon JG, Shaw AR, Dinarello CA, Reichlin S (1990) Immunoreactive interleukin-1β localization in the rat forebrain. *Brain Res* 514: 135–140

15 Sheeran P, Hall GM (1997) Cytokines in anaesthesia. *Brit J Anaes* 78: 201–219

16 Rotshenker S, Aamar S, and Barak V (1992) Interleukin-1 activity in lesioned peripheral nerve. *J Neuroimmunol* 39: 75–80

17 Watkins LR, Wiertelak EP, Goehler LE, Smith KP, Martin D, Maier SF (1994) Characterization of cytokine-induced hyperalgesia. *Brain Res* 654: 15–26

18 Oka T, Aou S, Hori T (1993) Intracerebroventricular injection of interleukin-1β induces hyperalgesia in rats. *Brain Res* 624: 61–68

19 Oka T, Aou S, Hori T (1994) Intracerebroventricular injection of interleukin-1β enhances nociceptive neuronal responses of trigeminal nucleus caudalis in rats. *Brain Res* 656: 236–244

20 Oka T, Oka K, Hosoi M, Aou S, Hori T (1995) The opposing effects of interleukin-1β microinjected into the preoptic hypothalamus on nociceptive behavior in rats. *Brain Res* 700: 271–278

21 Won C, Park HJ, Shin HC (1995) Interleukin-1β facilitates afferent sensory transmission in the primary somatosensory cortex of anesthestized rats. *Neurosci Letters* 201: 255–258

22 Patterson PH, Nawa H (1993) Neuronal differentiation factors/cytokines and synaptic plasticity. *Cell* 72: 123–137

23 Taga T (1996) gp130, a shared signal transducing receptor component for hematopoietic and neuropoietic cytokines. *J Neurochem* 67: 1–10

24 Kiefer R, Lindholm, D, Kreutzberg, G (1993) Interleukin-6 and transforming growth factor-β1 mRNAs are induced in rat facial nucleus following motorneuron axotomy. *Eur J Neurosci* 5: 775–781

25 Murphy PG, Grodin J, Altares M, Richardson PM (1995) Induction of interleukin-6 in axotomized sensory neurons. *J Neurosci* 15: 5130–5138

26 Bolin LM, Verity AN, Silver JE, Shooter EM, Abrams JS (1995) Interleukin-6 production in schwann cells and induction in sciatic nerve injury. *J Neurochem* 64: 850–858

27 Frei K, Malipiero UV, Leist TP, Zinkernagel RM, Schwab ME, Fontana A (1989) On the cellular source and function of interleukin-6 produced by the central nervous system. *Eur J Immunol* 19: 689–694

28 Le J, Vilcek J (1989) Interleukin-6: a multifunctional cytokine regulating immune reactions and the acute phase protein response. *Lab Invest* 61: 588–602

29 Fattori E, Lazzaro D, Musiani P, Modesti A, Alonzi T, Ciliberto G (1995) IL-6 expres-

sion in neurons of transgenic mice causes reactive astrocytosis and increase ramified microglial cells but no neuronal damage. *Eur J Neurosci* 7: 2441–2449

30 DeLeo JA and RW Colburn (1996) The role of cytokines in nociception and chronic pain. In: Weinstein J, Gordon S (eds): *Low back pain: A scientific and clinical overview.* American Academy of Orthopaedic Surgeons, Illinois, 163–186

31 Oka T, Oka K, Hosoi M, Hori T (1995) Intracerebroventricular injection of interleukin-6 induces thermal hyperalgesia in rats. *Brain Res* 692: 123–128

32 DeLeo JA, Colburn RW, Nichols M, Malhotra A (1996) Interleukin (IL)-6 mediated hyperalgesia/alloydnia and increased spinal IL-6 in a mononeuropathy model in the rat. *J Interferon and Cytokine Res* 16: 695–700

33 Qui Z, Parson KL, Gruol DL (1995) Interleukin-6 selectively enhances the intracellular calcium response to NMDA in developing CNS neurons. *J Neurosci* 15: 6688–6699

34 Meller ST, Gebhart GF (1993) Nitric oxide (NO) and nociceptive processing in the spinal cord. *Pain* 52: 127–136

35 Davar G, Jama A, Deykin A, Vos B, Maciewicz R (1991) MK-801 blocks the development of thermal hyperalgesia in a rat model of experimental painful neuropathy. *Brain Res* 553: 327–330

36 Price DD, Mao J, Frenk H, Mayer DJ (1994) The N-methyl-D-aspartate receptor antagonist dextromethorphan selectively reduces temporal summation of second pain in man. *Pain* 59: 165–174.

37 Beutler B, Greenwald D, Hulmes JD, Chang M, Pan YC, Mathison J, Ulevitch R, Cerami A (1985) Identity of tumour necrosis factor and the macrophage-secreted factor cachectin. *Nature* 316: 552–554

38 Carswell EA, Old LJ, Kassel RL, Green S, Fiore N, Williamson B (1975) An endotoxin-induced serum factor that causes necrosis of tumors. *Proc Natl Acad Sci* 72: 3666–3669

39 Tsujimoto M, Vilcek J (1986) Tumor necrosis factor receptors in HeLa cells and their regulation by interferon-gamma. *J Biol Chem* 261: 5384–5388

40 Smith CA, Davis T, Anderson D (1990) A receptor for tumor necrosis factor defines an unusual family of cellular and viral proteins. *Science* 248: 1019–1023

41 Loetscher H, Pan YC, Lahm HW (1990) Molecular cloning and expression of the human 55 kd tumor necrosis factor receptor. *Cell* 61: 351–359

42 Englemann H, Aderka D, Rubinstein M, Rotman D, Wallach D (1989) A tumor necrosis factor-binding protein purified to homogeneity from human urine protects cells from tumor necrosis factor toxicity. *J Biol Chem* 264: 11974–11980

43 Olsson I, Lantz M, Nilsson E (1989) Isolation and characterization of a tumor necrosis factor binding protein from urine. *Eur J Haematol* 42: 270–275

44 Moreland LW, Baumgartner SW, Schiff MH, Tindall EA, Fleischmann RM, Weaver AL, Ettlinger RE, Cohen S, Koopman WJ, Mohler K et al (1997) Treatment of rheumatoid arthritis with a recombinant human tumor necrosis factor receptor (p75)-Fc fusion protein. *New Eng J Med* 337: 141–147

45 Koller H, Thiem K, Siebler M (1996) Tumour necrosis factor-α increases intracellular Ca^{2+} and induces a depolarization in cultured astroglial cells. *Brain* 119: 2021–2027

46   Fine SM, Angel RA, Perry SW, Epstein LF, Rothstein JD, Dewhurst S, Gelbard HA
     (1996) Tumor necrosis factor-α inhibits glutamate uptake by primary human astrocytes.
     J Biol Chem 271(26): 15303–15306

47   Ding M, Hart RP, Jonakait FM (1995) Tumor necrosis factor-α induces substance P in
     sympathetic ganglia through sequential induction of Interleukin-1 and Leukemia
     Inhibitory Factor. *J Neurobiol* 28: 445–454

48   DeLeo JA, Colburn RW, Rickman AJ (1997) Cytokine and growth factor immunohis-
     tochemical spinal profiles in two animal models of mononeuropathy. *Brain Res* 759:
     50–57

49   Hickey, WF, Kimura H (1988) Perivascular microglia are bone marrow derived and pre-
     sent antigen *in vivo*. *Science* 239: 290–292

50   Streit WJ, and Kincaid-Colton CA (1995) The brain's immune system. *Scientific Amer*
     Nov: 54–61

51   Meller ST, Dykstra C, Grsybicki, Murphy S, Gebhart GF (1994) The possible role of glia
     in nociceptive processing and hyperalgesia in the spinal cord of the rat. *Neuropharm* 33:
     1471–1478

52   Garrison CJ, Dougherty PM, Kajander KC, Carlton SM (1991) Staining of glial fibril-
     lary acidic protein (GFAP) in lumbar spinal cord increases following a sciatic nerve con-
     striction injury. *Brain Res* 565: 1–7

53   Hajos F, Csillik B, Knyihar-Csillik E (1990) Alterations in glial fibrillary acidic protein
     immunoreactivity in the upper dorsal horn of the rat spinal cord in the course of trans-
     ganglionic atrophy and regenerative proliferation. *Neurosci Lett* 17: 8–13

54   Tetzlaff W, Graeber MB, Bisby MA, Kreutzberg GW (1988) Increased glial fibrillary
     protein synthesis in astrocytes during retrograde reaction of the rat facial nucleus. *Glia*
     1: 90–95

55   Norris JG, Benveniste EN (1993) Interleukin-6 production by astrocytes: Induction by
     the neurotransmitter norepinephrine. *J Neurosci* 45:137–146

56   Chung JM, Leem JW, Kim SH (1992) Somatic afferent fibers which continuously dis-
     charge after being isolated from their receptors. *Brain Res* 599: 29–33

57   Korenman EMD, Devor M (1981) Ectopic adrenergic sensitivity in damaged peripheral
     nerve axons in the rat. *Exp Neurol* 72: 63–81.

58   McLachlan EM, Janig W, Devor M, Michaelis M (1993) Peripheral nerve injury triggers
     noradrenergic sprouting within the dorsal root ganglia. *Nature* 363: 543–545

59   Sato J, Perl ER (1993) Adrenergic excitation of cutaneous pain receptors induced by
     peripheral nerve injury. *Science* 251:1608–1610

60   Ventimiglia R, Green MI, Geller HM (1987) Localization of β-adrenergic receptors on
     differentiated cells of the central nervous system in culture. *Proc Natl Acad Sci* 84:
     5073–5077

61   Furukawa S, Furukawa Y, Satoyoshi E, Hayashi K (1987) Regulation of nerve growth
     factor synthesis/secretion by catecholamine in cultured mouse astroglial cells. *Biochem
     Biophys Res Commun* 147: 1048–1054

62   Frohman EM, Vayuvegula B, van den Noort S, Gupta S (1988) Norepinephrine inhibits

gamma-interferon-induced MHC class II (Ia) antigen expression on cultured brain astrocytes. *J Neuroimmunol* 17: 89–101

63 Kashiba H, Senba E, Kawai Y, Ueda Y, Tohyama (1992) Axonal blockade induces the expression of vasoactive intestinal peptide and galanin in rat dorsal root ganglion neurons. *Brain Res* 577: 19–28

64 Sontheimer H, Black JA, Waxman SG (1996) Voltage-gated Na$^+$ channels in glia: properties and possible functions. *Trends Neurosci* 19: 325–331

65 Steinhauser C, Gallo V (1996) News on glutamate receptors in glial cells. *Trends Neurosci* 19: 339–345

66 Glabinshi AR, Balasingam V, Tani M, Kunket SL, Strieter RM, Yong VW, Ransohoff RM (1996) Chemokine monocyte chemoattractant protein-1 is expressed by astrocytes after mechanical injury to the brain. *J Immunol* 156: 4363–4368

67 Hurwitz AA, Lyman WD, Berman JW (1995) Tumor necrosis factor alpha and transforming growth factor beta upregulate astrocyte expression of monocyte chemoattractant protein-1. *J Neuroimmunol* 57: 193–198

68 Garrison CJ, Dougherty PM, Carlton SM (1994) GFAP expression in lumbar spinal cord of naive and neuropathic rats treated with MK-801. *Exp Neurol* 129: 237–243

69 Watkins LR, Marin D, Ulrich P, Tracey KJ, Maier SF (1997) Evidence for the involvement of spinal cord glia in subcutaneous formalin induced hyperalgesia in the rat. *Pain* 71: 225–235

70 Xiao WH, Wagner R, Myers RR, Sorkin LS (1996) TNF-α applied to the sciatic nerve trunk elicits background firing in nociceptive primary afferent fibers. *8th World Congress on Pain*. Vancouver, BC, Canada

71 Wagner R, Myers RR (1996) Endoneurial injection of TNF alpha produces neuropathic behaviors. *Neuro Report* 7: 2897–2901

72 Bennett GJ, Laird JMA (1992) Central changes contributing to neuropathic hyperalgesia. In: Willis, Jr. WD (ed): *Hyperalgesia and allodynia*. Raven Press, New York, 305–310

73 Wagner R, DeLeo JA, Coombs DW, Colburn RW, Willenbring S, Fromm C (1993) Spinal dynorphin bilaterally increases in a rat neuropathic pain model. *Brain Res* 629: 323–326

74 Wall PD (1983) Alterations in the central nervous system after deafferentation: Connectivity control. In: Bonica J (ed): *Advances in pain research and therapy*. Raven Press, New York, 677–689

75 Lewin GR, Rueff A, Mendell LM (1994) Peripheral and central mechanisms of NGF-induced hyperalgesia. *Eur J Neurosci* 6: 1903–1912

76 Strijbos P, Rothwell NJ (1995) Interleukin-1β attenuates excitatory amino acid-induced neurodegeneration *in vitro*: involvement of nerve growth factor. *J Neurosci* 15: 3468–3474

77 Lewin GR, Mendell LM (1993) Nerve growth factor and nociception. *TINS* 16: 353–365

Brain cytokines and pain

Takakazu Oka[1,2] and Tetsuro Hori[2]

[1]Department of Psychosomatic Medicine, Kyushu University, Faculty of Medicine, Fukuoka 812-8582, Japan; [2]Department of Physiology, Kyushu University, Faculty of Medicine, Fukuoka 812-8582, Japan

Introduction

Proinflammatory cytokines such as interleukin-1 (IL-1), interleukin-6 (IL-6) and tumor necrosis factor-α (TNFα) are well known to be involved in local manifestation of inflammation in response to local cellular injury, e.g. edema, migration of immunocompetent cells, local hyperthermia and hyperalgesia. These cytokines, when given peripherally, induce such inflammatory responses at local sites, and local hyperalgesia is caused by the sensitizing effects of cytokines on polymodal receptors [1, 2].

Besides their peripheral origins, these cytokines are also produced in the brain by astrocytes, microglial cells, endothelial cells, meningeal macrophages and probably also by neurons (reviewed in [3]). The synthesis of the cytokines in the brain has been substantiated by increases in both their activities and their gene expression after peripheral administrations of endotoxin [4–8], formalin [9], and during restraint stress [10], as well as during pathological processes (cerebral ischemia, bacterial infection) within the central nervous system (CNS). Like the cytokines, receptors for these cytokines and the binding sites have been widely described in the CNS (reviewed in [11]). Brain-derived cytokines cause diverse effects on the homeostatic functions controlled in the hypothalamus, such as thermoregulation, sleep, feeding, neuroendocrine secretion, autonomic nervous activities and peripheral immune reactivities [11–15]. These responses are almost identical with "sickness symptoms" observed during peripheral infection. Recent studies, including ours, have revealed that central injections of these cytokines may modulate nociception [16–26]. This review will provide evidence for pain modulatory actions of brain-derived cytokines in the hypothalamus and neighboring basal forebrain, discuss how the pain modulatory actions are related to prostaglandin E_2 (PGE_2), a secondary signal substance of proinflammatory cytokines, and propose a possible role for the pain-modulatory actions of central cytokines for the host during infection.

Cytokines and Pain, edited by Linda R. Watkins and Steven F. Maier
© 1999 Birkhäuser Verlag Basel/Switzerland

Effects of i.c.v. injection of IL-1 on nociception: behavioral study

The reports on the effects of intracerebroventricular (i.c.v.) or intracisternal (i.c.s.) injection of IL-1α and IL-1β on nociceptive behaviors are controversial; they have been reported to either decrease [16, 17], increase [18, 20], or not change [26] pain sensitivity in rats and mice (Tab. 1). Such different results could be explained by the differences in the experimental protocols such as the dose and the species of IL-1 used, the method of measuring pain responsivity, and the time schedule of observation. Furthermore, it should be noted that the altered nociceptive behaviors could reflect secondary effects of IL-1-induced responses such as fever and decreased vigilance on the behaviors [18]. Therefore, we tested the effects of i.c.v. injection of IL-1β in a wide range of doses (1 pg/kg–1 μg/kg, ca. 325 fg–325 ng/rat) on nociception both electrophysiologically as well as behaviorally [18, 19].

First, we observed the nociceptive behavioral responses, as assessed by the hot-plate test, after an i.c.v. injection of IL-1β. We injected recombinant human IL-1β (rhIL-1β) at doses of 1 pg/kg to 1 μg/kg (ca. 325 fg–325 ng/rat) into the lateral cerebroventricle of male Wistar rats weighing 300–350 g, and observed the changes in the paw-withdrawal latency after being placed on a hot plate (Fig. 1A and B) [18]. The paw-withdrawal latency significantly reduced after i.c.v. injections of rhIL-1β (10 pg/kg–1 ng/kg, ca. 3.25 pg–325 pg), suggesting hyperalgesia. The maximal response was obtained after injection of rhIL-1β at 100 pg/kg (32.5 pg). The reduction of paw-withdrawal latency began to appear 5 min after injection, reached a peak within 30 min and then slowly returned to the baseline level within 120 min. When the amount of rhIL-1β was increased over 1 ng/kg (up to 1 μg/kg = ca. 325 ng) or decreased to 1 pg/kg (ca.325 fg), the paw-withdrawal latency did not change. Although i.c.v. injection of rhIL-1β at 100 ng/kg (ca. 32.5 ng) raised the colonic temperature (T_{co}) by about 0.6° C 30 min after injection, that of rhIL-1β at 1 ng/kg (ca. 325 pg) had no effect. The rhIL-1β-induced hyperalgesic behavior was completely abolished by i.c.v. pretreatment with either IL-1 receptor antagonist (IL-1Ra) at 10 and 100 ng/kg (ca. 3.25 and 32.5 ng), sodium salicylate (a cyclooxygenase inhibitor) at 100 ng/kg (ca. 32.5 ng), diclofenac (a cyclooxygenase inhibitor) at 1 ng/kg (ca. 325 pg) or the neuropeptide α-melanocyte-stimulating hormone (αMSH), a potent   inhibitor of proinflammatory cytokines [27, 28], at 10 and 100 ng/kg (ca. 3.25 and 32.5 ng). Thus, an i.c.v. injection of small, non-pyrogenic doses of rhIL-1β (10 pg/kg–1 ng/kg = ca. 3.25–325 pg) may induce hyperalgesia 5-60 min after injection via a receptor-mediated, eicosanoid-dependent, αMSH-sensitive process in the rat. The receptor mediation and eicosanoids dependency in i.c.v. IL-1β-induced hyperalgesia have been recently confirmed [25].

The hyperalgesia after i.c.v. injection of rhIL-1β does not agree with those of two previous reports which demonstrated analgesia after central injection of rhIL-1α in mice [16, 29] and rats [17]. The discrepancy might be explained by the different types of IL-1 used. In fact, several studies have pointed out the difference in the cen-

Table 1 - Effects of i.c.v. injection of cytokines on nociception.

Cytokine	Effect	Dose	Duration	Animal	Method	Possible involvement	Other effects	Ref.
IL-1β	Hyperalgesia	3 pg–0.3 ng	5–60 min	Rat	Hot-plate test	IL-1 receptor, PGs		[18]
	Hyperalgesia	3 pg–0.3 ng	5–60 min	Rat	Recording of WDR neuron	IL-1 receptor, PGs		[19]
	Hyperalgesia	5–50 ng	15–55 min	Rat	Tail-flick test			[20]
	No effect	125–2000 U (= 0.25–4 ng)		Rat	Cold-water tail-flick test, Hot-plate test		fever	[26]
	Biphasic Hyperalgesia	10–100 pg	60–180 min	Rat	Paw-pressure test	IL-1 receptor, PGs, CRF		[25]
	Analgesia	1–10 ng	120–180 min			IL-1 receptor, CRF	fever	
IL-1α	Analgesia	48 ng/kg*	5–20 min	Mouse	Writhing test			[16]
		1 ng		Mouse	Writhing test	peripheral CRF		[29]
	Analgesia	2.5–15 ng	3–5 min	Rat	Hot-plate test			[17]
		5 ng	3 min	Rat	Hot-plate test			[35]
	No effect	250–1000 U (= 2.5–10 ng)		Rat	Cold-water tail-flick test, Hot-plate test	central CRF and NA	fever	[26]
IL-6	Hyperalgesia	0.3–300 ng	15–30 min	Rat	Hot-plate test	PGs		[21]
TNFα	Analgesia	1–3.5 ng	3–5 min	Rat	Hot-plate test	IL-1	decreased locomotion	[17]
	Hyperalgesia	10 pg–1 ng**	60 min	Rat	Plantar test	IL-1, PGs		[24]
IFNα	Analgesia	250–500 U***	5 min	Mouse	Hot-plate test	opioids		[53]
	Analgesia	15000 U		rat	Cold-water tail-flick test			[26]

*50% inhibition in 20 g mice. **Time of the maximal effect. ***10^4 U/mg protein.

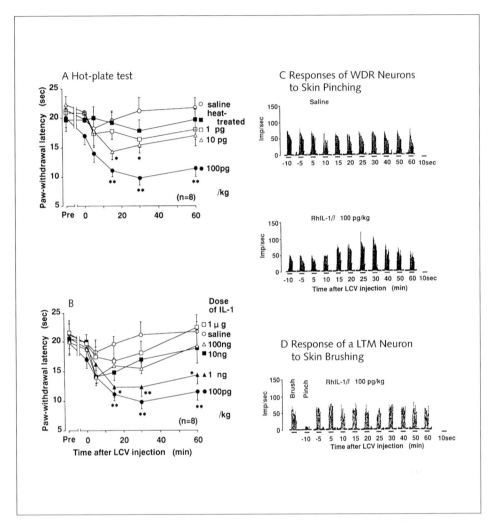

Figure 1

A and B; Effects of lateral cerebroventricular (LCV) injection of rhIL-1β on nociception as assessed by a hot-plate test. Rats weighing 300–350 g were injected with rhIL-1β at 1 pg/kg (□, A), 10 pg/kg (△, A), 100 pg/kg (●), 1 ng/kg (▲), 10 ng/kg (■, B), 100 ng/kg (△, B) or 1 μg/kg (□, B) or heat-inactivated rhIL-1β at 100 pg/kg (■, A), or saline (○). Each point represents mean ± S.E.M. Symbols adjacent to points represent the level of significance when compared with saline-injected controls. *p < 0.05; **p < 0.01. C; Changes in responses of WDR neurons to noxious pinching after LCV injection of saline or rhIL-1β at 100 pg/kg. D; Changes in the response of a LTM neuron to brushing after LCV injection of rhIL-1β at 100 pg/kg. Noxious pinching and brushing were applied during the underlined 10 sec periods. From [18, 19].

tral actions between IL-1α and IL-1β, e.g. the involvement of different mechanisms for the development of fever [30], different potency in producing adrenocorti-cotropic hormone (ACTH) [31] and PGE$_2$ [32], and different affinity for receptors in the brain [33]. However, Adams and colleagues [26] made an extensive study using two different methods (cold-water tail flick test and hot-plate test) to observe nociception and also repeated one of the previous studies [17] (same species/strain of animals, pain responsivity assay, dose range of rhIL-1α), but they failed to observe analgesia. They criticized the method of analgesic assay [16, 17] and the method of data analysis [17] employed in the previous studies as possible causes for discrepancy. Adams et al. [26] observed no analgesia and no hyperalgesia after i.c.v. injection of rhIL-1α (250–1000 U = ca. 2.5–10 ng) and rhIL-1β (125–2000 U = ca. 250 pg–4 ng). If the rhIL-1β they used has the same potency as that we used, their lowest dose of rhIL-1β corresponds roughly to the highest dose with which we observed a decrease in the nociceptive threshold as assessed by the hot-plate test.

On the other hand, hyperalgesia, as assessed by the tail-flick test, has recently been described after i.c.v. administration of rhIL-1β at 5 and 50 ng in the rat [20]. If their rhIL-1β, once again, has the same potency as ours, these doses of rhIL-1β would be expected not to alter T$_{co}$ (5 ng) or to raise T$_{co}$ by less than 1° C (50 ng), according to our study [18]. Another recent report has demonstrated a biphasic effect on mechanical nociception depending on the dose of i.c.v. rhIL-1β [25], i.e. hyperalgesia by rhIL-1β at non-pyrogenic doses (10–100 pg) was observed 60–180 min after injection and analgesia by that of pyrogenic doses (1–10 ng) was seen 120–180 min after injection. Although there are some differences among the results, these studies (including our own) indicate that i.c.v. injection of rhIL-1β at subpy-rogenic doses induces an increase in nociception to, at least, thermal and mechani-cal stimuli. On the other hand, there is still no general consensus for the analgesia seen after i.c.v. injection of IL-1 due to the divergent results, i.e. a rapid and tran-sient (3–5 min) analgesia [17], an extremely delayed analgesia (120–180 min) [25] or no analgesia [26].

It is well known that many IL-1β-induced responses are mediated via the neu-ropeptide corticotropin releasing factor (CRF) in the brain. However, it has not yet been settled as to whether the brain CRF system constitutes an essential component for the development of i.c.v. IL-1β-induced modulation of pain. In our study, the i.c.v. rhIL-1β (100 pg/kg, ca. 32.5 pg)-induced hyperalgesia was not affected by pre-treatment with α-helical CRF$_{9-41}$ (αhCRF, a CRF antagonist) at a dose of 100 ng/kg (ca. 32.5 ng), a dose that was previously shown to completely block the excitation of splenic sympathetic activity using the same amount of rhIL-1β [34]. By contrast, it was shown that similar pretreatment with αhCRF at 1 µg, which was about 31 times higher than that in our study, completely blocked both the hyperalgesic and analgesic effects of IL-1β [25]. As for the IL-1α-induced anti-nociception, one report [35] suggested that it was mediated by central CRF, whereas another study indicat-ed the involvement of peripheral, as opposed to central, CRF [29].

Effects of i.c.v. injection of IL-1 on nociception: electrophysiological study

Any behavioral methods for the measurement of nociceptive threshold, as was discussed in the introduction, are possibly contaminated by changes in non-nociceptive functions after cytokine administration. Therefore, it is imperative to obtain the electrophysiological evidence showing that similar doses of IL-1β may actually affect the nociceptive system. We investigated the effects of i.c.v. injection of IL-1β (1 pg/kg–1 μg/kg, ca. 325 fg–325 ng/rat) on the nociceptive responses of wide dynamic range (WDR) neurons in the trigeminal nucleus caudalis in the urethane-anesthetized rats [19] (Fig. 1C). The WDR neurons, along with the nociceptive specific neurons, may relay somatosensory signals from the cutaneous nociceptors to the thalamic nuclei. Noxious pinching stimuli were applied to the receptive field of the rat's face for a period of 10 sec at the scheduled times. An i.c.v. injection of rhIL-1β at 100 pg/kg (32.5 pg) enhanced the nociceptive responses of 10 of 13 (77%) WDR neurons tested, whereas physiological saline did not affect them. The maximal enhancement ($207 \pm 21\%$, n=10) was obtained 25 min after injection of rhIL-1β at 100 pg/kg (ca. 32.5 pg). RhIL-1β at 10 pg/kg (ca.3.25 pg) and 1 ng/kg (ca. 325 pg) also enhanced the responses of a similar population (67%) of WDR neurons, but the enhancing effects were smaller than that of rhIL-1β at 100 pg/kg (ca. 32.5 pg). The other doses of rhIL-1β had no significant effect on the neuronal responses. RhIL-1β (100 pg/kg = ca. 32.5 pg)-induced enhancement of the responses of WDR neurons to noxious stimuli was completely inhibited by i.c.v. pretreatment with IL-1Ra and sodium salicylate. These electrophysiological findings conform well with our results of behavioral studies [18] in terms of effective doses of IL-1β, time course, receptor mediation, and eicosanoid dependency. Furthermore, the inability to alter the nociceptive responses of WDR neurons by rhIL-1β between 10 ng/kg (ca. 3.25 ng) and 1 μg/kg (ca. 325 ng) is consistent with the observation of no changes in nociceptive behaviors at these doses [18, 26].

Low threshold mechanoreceptive (LTM) neurons in the trigeminal nucleus caudalis, which is known to relay cutaneous tactile signals to the CNS by responding only to innocuous mechanical stimuli, did not change their responsiveness to skin brushing after i.c.v. injection of rhIL-1β at 100 pg/kg (ca. 32.5 pg) (Fig. 1D). It thus appears that the enhancing effect of rhIL-1β on the responsiveness of somatosensory neurons in the trigeminal nucleus caudalis is modality specific.

Brain sites where IL-1 acts to modulate nociception

In order to determine the sites in the brain where IL-1 acts to induce hyperalgesia, we investigated nociceptive behaviors on the hot-plate after microinjection of rhIL-1β (0.5 pg/kg–2 ng/kg = ca. 163 fg–650 pg/rat) into different sites in the hypothalamus and neighboring basal forebrain of rats [22]. A microinjection of rhIL-1β between 5 and 50 pg/kg (ca. 1.63 pg–16.3 pg) into the medial part of the preoptic area (MPO) decreased the paw-withdrawal latency, producing a maximal response at a dose of 20 pg/kg (ca. 6.5 pg) (Fig. 2A and B). At this dose of rhIL-1β, the paw-withdrawal latency began to decrease 15 min after injection, reached a minimum at 30 min and gradually returned to the baseline latency. The other doses of rhIL-1β tested had no significant effect. The hyperalgesic response was also obtained after injection of rhIL-1β at 20 pg/kg (ca. 6.5 pg) into the lateral part of the preoptic area (LPO), the median preoptic nucleus (MnPO) and the diagonal band of Broca (DBB), but not after injection into the paraventricular nucleus (PVN), the lateral hypothalamic area (LH), and the septal nucleus (Fig. 3). Although the MPO is known to be sensitive to microinjected IL-1β, resulting in a raise in body temperature, microinjection of rhIL-1β at 20 pg/kg (ca. 6.5 pg), the dose which induced a maximal degree of hyperalgesia, into the MPO had no effect on T_{co} (Fig. 2C). In contrast, microinjection of rhIL-1β at 20 pg/kg (ca. 6.5 pg) and 50 pg/kg (ca. 16.25 pg) into the ventromedial hypothalamus (VMH) prolonged the paw-withdrawal latency 5 min and 5–10 min after injection, respectively, suggesting analgesia (Fig. 2D and E). When the doses of rhIL-1β into the VMH increased to 200 pg/kg (ca. 65 pg) and 2 ng/kg (ca. 650 pg) or decreased to 5 pg/kg (ca. 1.63 pg), the paw-withdrawal latency did not change significantly. In another study [23], nociception was examined only 60 min after microinjection of rhIL-1β (5 ng, a pyrogenic dose when given into the MPO) into the discrete sites in the diencephalon of rats. RhIL-1β (5 ng) had hyperalgesic effects in the PVN and analgesic effects in the centro-medial and gelatinous nuclei of the thalamus. The microinjection of rhIL-1β (5 ng) into neither the MPO nor the VMH had any effect on nociception, which is in line with our results (Tab. 2).

Table 2 - Brain sites where IL-1β acts to modulate nociception revealed by the microinjection studies

Effect	Brain sites	Dose of IL-1β	Ref.
hyperalgesia	hypothalamus		
	preoptic area	5–50 pg/kg[*]	[22]
	paraventricular nucleus	5 ng	[23]
	diagonal band of Broca	20 pg/kg[*]	[22]
analgesia	hypothalamus		
	ventromedial hypothalamus	20–50 pg/kg[*]	[22]
	thalamus		
	centro-medial nucleus	5 ng	[23]
	gelatinous nucleus	5 ng	[23]

[*]Rats weighing 320–350 g. Taken from [22] and [23].

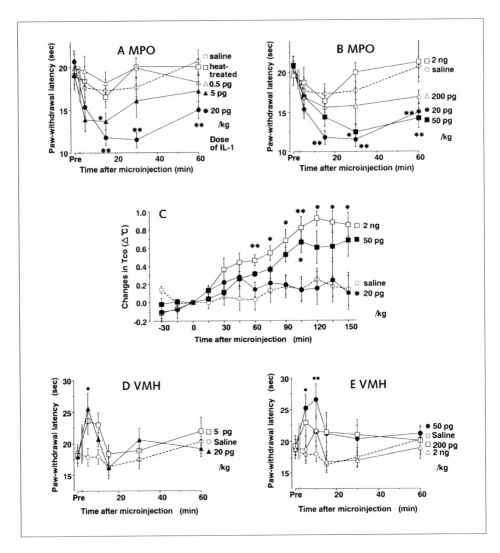

Figure 2

The opposing effects of rhIL-1β microinjected into the medial part of the preoptic area (MPO; A-C) and the ventromedial hypothalamus (VMH; D and E) on nociception as assessed by a hot-plate test. In A-C, rats weighing 320–350 g were injected with rhIL-1β at 0.5 pg/kg (△, A), 5 pg/kg (▲), 20 pg/kg (●), 50 pg/kg (■), 200 pg/kg (△, B) or 2 ng/kg (□, B and C) or heat inactivated rhIL-1β at 20 pg/kg (□, A), or saline (○). In D and E, rats were injected with rhIL-1β at 5 pg/kg (□, D), 20 pg/kg (▲), 50 pg/kg (●), 200 pg/kg (□, E) or 2 ng/kg (△), or saline (○). n = 8–14. Each point represents mean ± S.E.M. Symbols adjacent to points represent significance when compared with saline-injected controls. *p < 0.05; **p < 0.01. From [22].

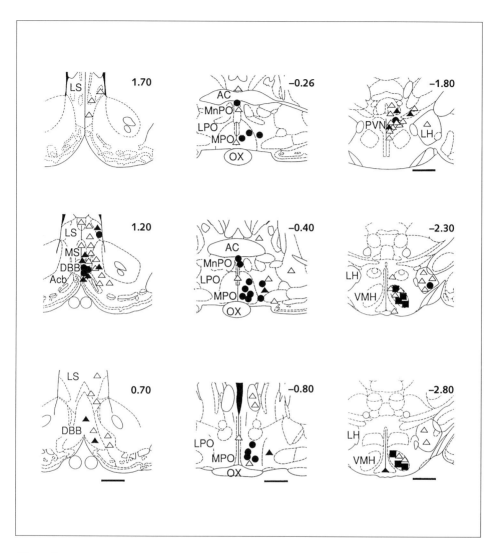

Figure 3

Brain sites where the microinjection of rhIL-1β at 20 pg/kg induce hyperalgesia (●,▲) and hypoalgesia (■). The magnitude of hyperalgesic and analgesic responses was expressed as the percentage of the maximal change in the paw-withdrawal latency to the baseline latency. ● ≤60%, 60% < ▲ ≤70%, 70% < △ <130%, ■ ≥130%. LS, lateral septal nucleus; MS, medial septal nucleus; DBB, diagonal band of Broca; Acb, accumbens nucleus; AC, anterior commissure; MnPO, median preoptic nucleus; MPO, medial part of the preoptic area; LPO, lateral part of the preoptic area; OX, optic chiasma; PVN, paraventricular nucleus; LH, lateral hypothalamic area; VMH, ventromedial hypothalamus. Bar=1mm. The numbers on the right of individual frontal sections indicate the distances in mm from bregma. From [22].

Despite the different time courses of the intraVMH rhIL-1β-induced analgesia (5–10 min) and the intraMPO rhIL-1β-induced hyperalgesia (15–60 min), both types of pain modulatory action of rhIL-1β were inhibited by the simultaneous injection of IL-1Ra or sodium salicylate (or diclofenac), suggesting that analgesia as well as hyperalgesia was receptor-mediated and eicosanoid-dependent. This is consistent with the electrophysiological findings showing the suppression of rhIL-1β-induced changes in the firing activity of MPO neurons by IL-1Ra [36] and sodium salicylate [37] and those of VMH neurons by sodium salicylate [12].

These findings indicate that brain IL-1β produces hyperalgesia and analgesia with different time courses depending on the amount and the site of its action in the hypothalamus and neighboring basal forebrain. This suggests that the altered nociceptive behavior observed after i.c.v. injection of rhIL-1β reflects the net result of hyperalgesic and analgesic responses with different characteristics and it might also reflect the difference in accessibility of i.c.v. injected rhIL-1β to its active sites. Conflicting findings on altered nociceptive behaviors after i.c.v. injection of rhIL-1β might be explained, at least partly, on the basis of these complicated factors.

Possible mechanisms of pain modulatory actions of IL-1β in the hypothalamus and neighboring basal forebrain

It is at present unknown how the altered activities of MPO and VMH neurons induced by IL-1β produce hyperalgesia and analgesia, respectively. One possible mechanism is that changes in the activity of hypothalamic neurons may affect the activities of neurons in the nuclei of the lower brainstem such as the periaqueductal grey matter (PAG) and the nucleus raphe magnus (NRM), which belong to the descending pain reducing system (DPRS). It has been demonstrated that electrical stimulation of the MPO produces analgesia as assessed by behavioral testing and the suppression of nociceptive neuronal responses in the trigeminal nucleus caudalis in the rat [38] and in the spinal dorsal horn in the cat [39]. The electrical stimulation of the VMH and the DBB also induces analgesia [39, 40] and the lesioning of VMH induces hyperalgesia [41]. It has been suggested that the analgesic effects of stimulation of MPO, DBB and VMH are mediated by the activation of the DPRS in the lower brainstem [38, 42]. In addition, direct neuronal connections have been histologically demonstrated from the MPO and adjacent nuclei to the PAG [43]. On the other hand, several electrophysiological studies have revealed that IL-1 predominantly decreases the firing rate of MPO neurons [36, 37, 44] and increases the activity of VMH neurons [12], respectively. Therefore, it is possible to suggest that the decreased activity of the MPO and the increased activity of the VMH by IL-1β actually suppresses and enhances the activity of the DPRS, respectively, thereby producing hyperalgesia and analgesia.

However, because of the complexity of the DPRS and the descending pain enhancing system recently proposed [45, 46], more complicated mechanisms which underlie the IL-1-induced modulation of pain might exist. Further studies are required to elucidate this issue.

Effects of other cytokines in the brain on nociception

We further investigated the effects of other proinflammatory cytokines such as rhIL-6 (30 pg–300 ng) and rhTNFα (1 pg–10 ng) on nociception in rats, both of which are known to be produced in the brain [6–8, 47–50].

RhIL-6 (300pg–300 ng) and rhTNFα (10 pg–1 ng) reduced the paw-withdrawal latency on a hot-plate 15–30 min and to radiant heat 60 min, respectively, after i.c.v. injection [21, 24]. All the doses of both cytokines were non-pyrogenic and non-somnogenic, except for rhIL-6 at 300 ng which produced a delayed rise in the T_{co} which started 70 min after injection. The increased nociceptive sensitivity, however, was observed 15 and 30 min after its injection when there was no change in T_{co}. The simultaneous i.c.v. injection of sodium salicylate and diclofenac blocked the hyperalgesic effects of rhIL-6 and rhTNFα, respectively, indicating the involvement of eicosanoid synthesis [51, 52]. Although IL-1Ra (i.c.v.) did not affect the rhIL-6-induced hyperalgesia, it abolished the rhTNFα-induced hyperalgesia. This suggests that the TNFα-induced hyperalgesia is mediated by the central action of IL-1, probably by its ability to induce IL-1 [52].

On the other hand, Bianchi et al. [17] reported that i.c.v. injection of recombinant murine TNFα (1–3.5 ng) induced a rapid and short-lasting (3–5 min after injection) analgesia as assessed by the hot-plate test. This analgesia was antagonized by anti-IL-1 antibodies, but not by indomethacin (a cyclooxygenase inhibitor), naloxone (an opioid antagonist), or anti-sera against β-endorphin, met-enkephalin and dynorphin.

Central administration of interferon-α (IFNα) has also been demonstrated to induce analgesia [26, 53]. This analgesia was inhibited by naloxone [53] like the other CNS responses to IFNα including catalepsy [53], fever [54], reduced cytotoxicity of splenic natural killer cells [15], and altered activities of hypothalamic neurons [12, 55]. This was taken to be mediated by its binding to opioid receptors [56].

Effects of central injection of PGE$_2$ and its agonists on nociception in the brain

Since an obligatory role of eicosanoid(s) was proposed in the pain modulatory effects of central IL-1, IL-6 and TNFα, we further investigated the effects of central administration of PGE$_2$ and its agonists on nociception, both behaviorally and electrophysiologically, in the rat. The reasons why we focused on PGE_2 among many eicosanoids were (1) that PGE_2 was assumed to be a principal mediator of IL-1-induced CNS-mediated actions such as fever [11] or ACTH release [57], (2) that IL-1β and IL-6 specifically increased the release of PGE_2 from rat hypothalamic explants *in vitro* [51], (3) that dense PGE_2 binding sites [58, 59] and the expression of PGE_2 receptor mRNA [60] were demonstrated in the hypothalamus, and (4) that there were many neurons in the MPO and adjacent regions which changed the firing rate after application of PGE_2 [61].

Our behavioral and electrophysiological studies [62, 63] revealed that PGE_2 in the brain induced a biphasic effect on nociception depending on the doses administered (Fig. 4). An i.c.v. injection of PGE_2 at low (non-pyrogenic) doses (10 pg/kg–10 ng/kg = ca. 3.25 pg–3.25 ng or ca. 9 fmol–9 pmol) induced a long-lasting (5–60 min after injection) hyperalgesia as assessed by the hot-plate test and a rapid, short-lasting (5 min) analgesia at a high (pyrogenic) dose (1 μg/kg = ca. 325 ng = ca. 900 pmol) in rats [62]. In accordance with this, an i.c.v. injection of PGE_2 at low doses (353 fg–3.53 pg = 1–10 fmol) enhanced the responses of the WDR neurons in the trigeminal nucleus to skin pinching 15–25 min after injection, whereas that of higher doses (35.3–353 ng = 100 pmol–1 nmol) suppressed them 5–15 min after injection in anesthetized rats [63]. The responses of LTM neurons to tactile stimuli were not affected by i.c.v. injection of PGE_2, indicating that the modulatory effect of PGE_2 on the responsiveness of somatosensory neurons is modality specific.

Pharmacological and molecular biological studies have demonstrated that PGE_2 (EP-) receptors are classified into four subtypes, i.e., EP_1, EP_2, EP_3 and EP_4 receptors, which activate or inhibit the different types of second messengers [64, 65]. Among the synthetic EP-receptor agonists, an i.c.v. injection of an EP_3 receptor agonist, M&B28767 (1 pg/kg–100 pg/kg = ca. 325 fg–32.5 pg = ca. 0.9 fmol–90 fmol), reduced the paw-withdrawal latency on a hot-plate 15–60 min after injection and enhanced the responses of WDR neurons to noxious stimuli [62, 66]. On the other hand, i.c.v. injection of an EP_1 receptor agonist, 17-phenyl-ω-trinor PGE_2 (50 μg/kg = ca.16.25 μg = ca. 42 nmol), prolonged the paw-withdrawal latency only 5 min after injection and suppressed the responses of WDR neurons with a similar time course [62, 66]. Furthermore, the PGE_2 (353 ng = ca. 1 nmol, i.c.v.)-induced analgesic effects observed neurophysiologically as well as behaviorally were inhibited by an EP_1 receptor antagonist, SC19220. An EP_2 receptor agonist, butaprost (1 pg/kg–100 μg/kg = ca. 325 fg–32.5 μg) had no effect on nociception. Therefore, these findings suggest that small amounts of PGE_2 induce a relatively long-lasting hyperalgesia through EP_3 receptors and large amounts of PGE_2 produces a rapid, short-lasting analgesia through EP_1 receptors in the brain.

We then microinjected PGE_2 and its receptor agonists into several sites in the rat brain and assessed the changes in nociception by the hot-plate test [67]. The

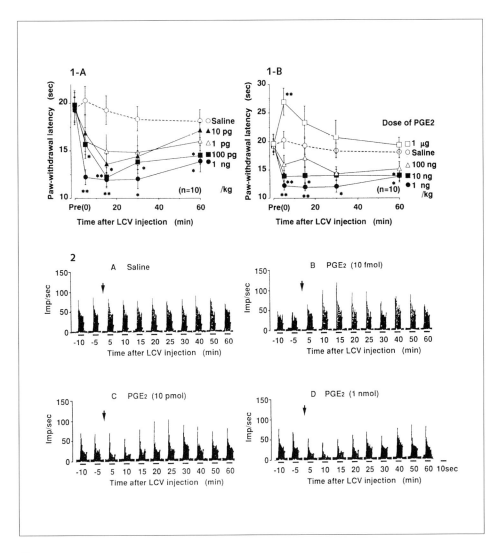

Figure 4

*1A and B; Effects of LCV injection of PGE$_2$ on nociception as assessed by a hot-plate test. Rats weighing 300–350 g were injected with PGE$_2$ at 1 pg/kg (△, A), 10 pg/kg (▲). 100 pg/kg (■, A), 1 ng/kg (●), 10 ng/kg (■, B), 100 ng/kg (△, B) or 1 μg/kg (□), or saline (○). Each point represents mean ± S.E.M. Symbols adjacent to points represent the level of significance when compared with saline-injected controls. *p < 0.05; **p < 0.01. 2A-D; Effects of LCV injection of physiological saline (A) and PGE$_2$ at 10 fmol (3.53 pg, B), 10 pmol (3.53 ng, C) and 1 nmol (353 ng, D) on the responses of the WDR neurons to noxious pinching stimuli. The WDR neurons shown in B, C, and D were classified as "increased", "biphasic, i.e., decrease followed by increase" and "decreased" neurons, respectively. From [62, 63].*

microinjection of low doses of PGE_2 (5–50 fg) and M&B28767 (0.05–5 fg) into the MPO reduced the paw-withdrawal latency in a U-shaped fashion in rats. The M&B28767-induced hyperalgesia was also obtained in the LPO, the MnPO, and the DBB. The microinjection of neither 17-phenyl-ω-trinor PGE_2 nor butaprost had any effect on nociception in these nuclei. On the other hand, the microinjection of PGE_2 (5–500 pg) and 17-phenyl-ω-trinor PGE_2 (500 pg) into the VMH prolonged the paw-withdrawal latency. The analgesia after intraVMH injection of PGE_2 was inhibited by the co-injection of SC19220 [our unpublished observation]. These findings suggest that PGE_2 at low concentrations induces hyperalgesia through EP_3 receptors in the MPO, LPO, MnPO and the DBB, whereas PGE_2 at high levels induces analgesia through EP_1 receptors in the VMH.

Although it has not been determined as to how the density and distribution of these EP receptors in the brain vary, *in situ* hybridization studies have demonstrated that the EP_3 receptor mRNA is much more abundant in the brain (including the MPO and the DBB) than the EP_1 receptor transcripts [60] and no EP_2 receptor mRNA is detectable in the brain [68]. The cloned mouse EP_3 receptors have a higher affinity to PGE_2 than the EP1 receptors [65]. Another question is why the hyperalgesic actions disappear at higher doses of PGE_2 and M&B28767. One possible explanation might be the desensitization of EP_3 receptors which occurs during exposure to high levels of PGE_2 [69]. Thus, the switching from hyperalgesia to analgesia with an increase in central PGE_2 occurs by changes in the EP receptors being stimulated. It is interesting that EP_1 receptors, but not other types of EP receptors, in the brain also mediate fever [70, 71] and activation of the splenic sympathetic nerve [72] by central PGE_2 given at high doses which produce analgesia.

Involvement of central cytokines in the development of hyperalgesia induced by peripheral administration of LPS and IL-1β

We observed that intraperitoneal (i.p.) injection of non-pyrogenic doses of rhIL-1β (10–100 ng/kg = ca. 3.25–32.5 ng) produced hyperalgesia as measured by the hot-plate test in rats [73]. The hyperalgesia (100 ng/kg = 32.5 ng, i.p.) was inhibited by i.c.v. pretreatment with diclofenac (1 ng) or αMSH (100 ng), both of which alone had no effect on nociception. These findings suggest that hyperalgesia induced by peripheral IL-1β may also be modulated by as yet unknown central mechanisms involving the synthesis of eicosanoids, an αMSH sensitive process, and probably the production of brain cytokines.

An i.p. injection of LPS (200 µg/kg) and lithium chloride (LiCl, 0.15 M) is also known to produce hyperalgesia, which is blocked by IL-1Ra, suggesting the mediation by IL-1 [74]. However, it is unknown whether the source of such IL-1 and the site(s) of its actions for the development of hyperalgesia are in the CNS or the peripheral tissues. Watkins and colleagues [45] have revealed that such sickness-inducing agents (i.p.) produce hyperalgesia by activating vagal afferents (rather than generating a blood-borne mediator), the neural signals of which eventually reach as yet undetermined brain site(s) rostral to the mid-mesencephalon, and, centrifugally, a descending pathway arising from the nucleus raphe magnus through the dorsolateral funiculus of the spinal cord.

An i.p. or intravenous injection of LPS increases the levels of IL-1β, IL-6 and TNFα and their mRNA in the brain [4–8, 50]. Subdiaphragmatic vagotomy blocks the LPS (i.p.)-induced expression of IL-1β mRNA in the mouse brain [75]. Furthermore, an i.p. injection of LPS also increases the expression of cyclooxygenase-2 (COX-2) and its mRNA in the brain [76]. Therefore, these observations suggest that such brain-derived cytokines and eicosanoid(s) are also involved in the hyperalgesia seen after i.p. injection of LPS. However, considering the rapid onset of hyperalgesia (5 min after LPS injection), the brain-derived cytokines [5, 50] and eicosanoid(s) [77] are unlikely to be responsible for, at least, the early phase of hyperalgesia after i.p. injection of LPS. Rather, they might contribute to the maintenance of the LPS hyperalgesia which lasts 55 min, the longest time of observation [45].

Conclusion

It is clear that PGE_2 is not the only signal molecule to mediate the central actions of IL-1, IL-6 and TNFα. It remains to be elucidated whether and how nociception may be modulated by other substances such as the other arachidonate metabolites and nitric oxide. In fact, it has been demonstrated that i.c.v. injection of PGD_2 and $PGF_{2\alpha}$ exhibit anti-nociceptive effects [78–80]. However, the characteristic pain modulatory effects of PGE_2 stated above are strikingly similar to those of the cytokines examined, particularly IL-1β, i.e., an opposite effect on nociception with different time courses depending on the dose administered and the site of injections in the hypothalamus. Therefore, the pain modulatory actions of IL-1β, IL-6 and TNFα in the hypothalamus may be mediated, at least partly, by PGE_2 locally released. We conclude that small amounts of IL-1β produce hyperalgesia via an action of PGE_2 on EP_3 receptors of neurons in the MPO region and large amounts of IL-1β induce analgesia via an action of PGE_2 on EP_1 receptors of neurons in the VMH area. The hyperalgesia induced by cytokines and PGE_2 at non-pyrogenic doses might explain systemic hyperalgesia clinically observed in the early phase of infectious diseases, and it would serve as a warning signal of infection before the development of typical sickness symptoms including fever, anorexia, sleepiness, neuroendocrine changes and sympathetic activation [81] (Fig. 5). The switching of nociceptive reactivity from hyperalgesia to analgesia which is accompanied by other sickness symptoms may reflect the changes in the strategy of the host for fighting microbial invasion as the disease progresses.

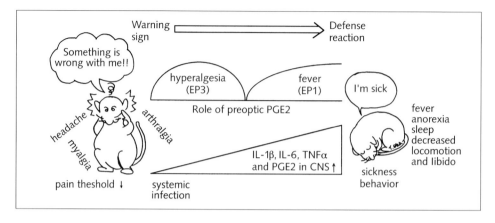

Figure 5
Physiological significance of brain cytokines-induced modulation of nociception.

Acknowledgements

This work was supported by Grant-in-Aid for General Scientific Research (No. 09557006 and No. 08877017 to T. Hori and No. 8473 to T. Oka) from the Ministry of Education, Science and Culture, Japan. These experiments were reviewed by the Committee of Ethics on Animal Experiments in the Faculty of Medicine, Kyushu University and was carried out under the control of the Guidelines for Animal Experiments of the Faculty of Medicine, Kyushu University and the Law (No.105) and Notification (No. 6) of the Government.

References

1   Cunha FQ, Poole S, Lorenzetti BB, Ferreira SH (1992) The pivotal role of tumor necrosis factor α in the development of inflammatory hyperalgesia. *Br J Pharmacol* 107: 660–664

2   Fukuoka H, Kawatani M, Hisamitsu T, Takeshige C (1994) Cutaneous hyperalgesia induced by peripheral injection of interleukin-1β in the rat. *Brain Res* 657: 133–140

3   Koening JI (1991) Presence of cytokines in the hypothalamic-pituitary axis. *Prog NeuroEndoImmunol* 4: 143–153

4   Clark BD, Bedrosian I, Schindler R, Cominelli F, Cannon JG, Shaw AR, Dinarello CA (1991) Detection of interleukin 1α and 1β in rabbit tissues during endotoxemia using sensitive radioimmunoassays. *J Appl Physiol* 71: 2412–2418

5   van Damm A-M, Brouns M, Louisse S, Berkenbosch F (1992) Appearance of interleukin-1 in macrophages and in ramified microglia in the brain of endotoxin-treated

rats: a pathway for the induction of non-specific symptoms of sickness? *Brain Res* 588: 291–296

6   Coceani F, Lees J, Mancilla J, Berlizario J, Dinarello CA (1993) Interleukin-6 and tumor necrosis factor in cerebrospinal fluid: Changes during pyrogen fever. *Brain Res* 612: 165–171

7   Klir JJ, Roth J, Szelenyi Z, McClellan JL, Kluger MJ (1993) Role of hypothalamic inter-leukin-6 and tumor necrosis factor-α in LPS fever in rat. *Am J Physiol* 265: R512–R517

8   Breder CD, Hazuka C, Ghayur T, Klug C, Huginin M, Yasuda K, Teng M, Saper CB (1994) Regional induction of tumor necrosis factor a expression in the mouse brain after systemic lipopolysaccharide administration. *Proc Natl Acad Sci USA* 91: 11393–11397

9   Yabuuchi K, Maruta E, Minami M, Satoh M (1996) Induction of interleukin-1β mRNA in the hypothalamus following subcutaneous injections of formalin into the rat hind paws. *Neurosci Lett* 207: 109–112

10   Minami M, Kuraishi Y, Yamaguchi T, Nakai S, Hirai Y, Satoh M (1991) Immobilization stress induces interleukin-1β mRNA in the rat hypothalamus. *Neurosci Lett* 123: 254–256

11   Faggioni R, Benigni F, Ghezzi P (1995) Proinflammatory cytokines as pathogenetic mediators in the central nervous system: brain-periphery connection. *Neuroim-munomodulation* 2: 2–15

12   Kuriyama K, Hori T, Mori T, Nakashima T (1990) Actions of interferon α and inter-leukin-1β on the glucose-responsive neurons in the ventromedial hypothalamus. *Brain Res Bull* 24: 803–810

13   Krueger JM, Toth LA, Floyd R, Fang J, Kapas L, Bredow S, Obal F (1994) Sleep, microbes and cytokines. *Neuroimmunomodulation* 1: 100–109

14   Hori T, Nakashima T, Take S, Kaizuka Y, Mori T, Katafuchi T (1991) Immune cytokines and regulation of body temperature, food intake and cellular immunity. *Brain Res Bull* 27: 309–313

15   Hori T, Katafuchi T, Take S, Shimizu N, Niijima A (1995) The autonomic nervous sys-tem as a communication channel between the brain and the immune system. *Neuroim-munomodulation* 2: 203–215

16   Nakamura H, Nakanishi K, Kita A, Kadokawa T (1988) Interleukin-1 induces analge-sia in mice by a central action. *Eur J Pharmacol* 149: 49– 54

17   Bianchi M, Sacerdote P, Ricciardi-Castagnoli P, Mantegazza P, Panerai AE (1992) Cen-tral effects of tumor necrosis factor-α and interleukin-1α on nociceptive thresholds and spontaneous locomotor activity. *Neurosci Lett* 148: 76–80

18   Oka T, Aou S, Hori T (1993) Intracerebroventricular injection of interleukin-1β induces hyperalgesia in rats. *Brain Res* 624: 61–68

19   Oka T, Aou S, Hori T (1994) Intracerebroventricular injection of interleukin-1β enhances nociceptive neuronal responses of the trigeminal nucleus caudalis in rats. *Brain Res* 656: 236–244

20   Watkins LR, Wiertelak EP, Goehler LE, Smith KP, Martin D, Maier SF (1994) Charac-terization of cytokine-induced hyperalgesia. *Brain Res* 654: 15–26

21 Oka T, Oka K, Hosoi M, Hori T (1995) Intracerebroventricular injection of interleukin-6 induces thermal hyperalgesia in rats. *Brain Res* 692: 123–128

22 Oka T, Oka K, Hosoi M, Aou S, Hori T (1995) The opposing effects of interleukin-1β microinjected into the preoptic hypothalamus and the ventromedial hypothalamus on nociceptive behavior in rats. *Brain Res* 700: 271–278

23 Sellami S, de Beaurepaire R (1995) Hypothalamic and thalamic sites of action of interleukin-1β on food intake, body temperature and pain sensitivity in the rat. *Brain Res* 694: 69–77

24 Oka T, Wakugawa Y, Hosoi M, Oka K, Hori T (1996) Intracerebroventricular injection of tumor necrosis factor-α induces thermal hyperalgesia in rats. *Neuroimmunomodulation* 3: 135–140

25 Yabuuchi K, Nishiyori A, Minami M, Satoh M (1996) Biphasic effects of intracerebroventricular interleukin-1β on mechanical nociception in the rat. *Eur J Pharmacol* 300: 59–65

26 Adams JU, Bussiere JL, Geller EB, Adler MW (1993) Pyrogenic doses of intracerebroventricular interleukin-1 did not induce analgesia in the rat hot-plate or cold-water tail flick tests. *Life Sci* 53: 1401–1409

27 Feng JD, Dao T, Lipton JM, Effects of preoptic microinjection of a-MSH on fever and normal temperature control in rabbits. *Brain Res Bull* 18: 473–477

28 Catania A, Lipton JM (1994) The neuropeptide alpha-melanocyte-stimulating hormone; a key component of neuroimmunomodulation. *Neuroimmunomodulation* 1: 93–99

29 Kita A, Imano K, Nakamura H (1993) Involvement of corticotropin-releasing factor in the antinociception produced by interleukin-1 in mice. *Eur J Pharmacol* 273: 317–322

30 Busbridge NJ, Dascombe MJ, Tilders FJH, van Oers JWAM, Linton EA, Rothwell NJ (1989) Central activation of thermogenesis and fever by interleukin-1β and interleukin-1α involves different mechanisms. *Biochem Biophys Res Commun* 162: 591–596

31 Uehara A, Gottshall PE, Dahl RK, Arimura A (1987) Stimulation of ACTH release by human interleukin-1β, but not by interleukin-1α, in conscious freely moving rats. *Biochem Biophys Res Commun* 146: 1286–1290

32 Katsuura G, Gottshall PE, Dahl RR, Arimura A (1989) Interleukin-1 beta increases prostaglandin E_2 in rat astrocyte cultures: modulatory effect of neuropeptides. *Endocrinology* 124: 3125–3127

33 Katsuura G, Gottshall PE, Arimura A (1988) Identification of a high-affinity receptor for interleukin-1 beta in rat brain. *Biochem Biophys Res Commun* 156: 61–67

34 Ichijo T, Katafuchi T, Hori T (1994) Central interleukin-1β enhances splenic sympathetic nerve activity in rats. *Brain Res Bull* 34: 547–553

35 Bianchi M, Panerai A (1995) CRH and the noradrenergic system mediate the antinociceptive effect of central interleukin-1α in the rat. *Brain Res Bull* 36: 113–117

36 Xin L, Blatteis CM (1992) Blockade by interleukin-1 receptor antagonist of IL-1β-induced neuronal activity in guinea pig preoptic area slices. *Brain Res* 569: 348–352

37 Hori T, Shibata M, Nakashima T, Yamasaki M, Asami A, Asami T, Koga H (1988)

Effects of interleukin-1 and arachidonate on the preoptic and anterior hypothalamic neurons. *Brain Res Bull* 20: 75–82

38   Mokha SS, Goldsmith GE, Hellon RF, Puri R (1987) Hypothalamic control of nocireceptive and other neurones in the marginal layer of the dorsal horn of the medulla (trigeminal nucleus caudalis) in the rat. *Exp Brain Res* 65: 427–436

39   Carstens E, MacKinnon JD, Guinan MJ (1982) Inhibition of spinal dorsal horn neuronal responses to noxious skin heating by medial preoptic and septal stimulation in the cat. *J Neurophysiol* 48: 981–991

40   Rhodes DL, Liebeskind JC (1978) Analgesia from rostral brain stem stimulation in the rat. *Brain Res* 143: 521–532

41   Vidal C, Jacob J (1980) The effect of medial hypothalamic lesions on pain control. *Brain Res* 199: 89–100

42   Takeshige C, Sato T, Mera T, Hisamitsu T, Fang J (1992) Descending pain inhibitory system involved in acupuncture analgesia. *Brain Res* Bull 29: 617–634

43   Rizvi TA, Ennis M, Shipley MT (1992) Reciprocal connections between the medial preoptic area and the midbrain periaqueductal gray in rat: a WGA-HRP and PHA-L study. *J Comp Neurol* 315: 1–15

44   Nakashima T, Hori T, Mori T, Kuriyama K, Mizuno K (1989) Recombinant human interleukin-1β alters the activity of preoptic thermosensitive neurons *in vitro*. *Brain Res* Bull 23: 209–213

45   Watkins LR, Wiertelak EP, Goehler LE, Mooney-Heiberger K, Martinez J, Furness L, Smith KP, Maier SF (1994) Neurocircuitry of illness-induced hyperalgesia. *Brain Res* 639: 283–299

46   Fields HL (1992) Is there a facilitatory component to central pain modulation. *Am Physiol Soc J* 1: 71–79

47   Aloisi F, Care A, Borsellino G, Gallo P, Rosa S, Bassani A, Cabibbo A, Testa U, Levi G, Peschle C (1992) Production of hemolymphopoietic cytokines (IL-6, IL-8, colony-stimulating factors) by normal human astrocytes in response to IL-1β and tumor necrosis factor-α. *J Immunol* 149: 2358–2366

48   Sawada M, Suzumura A, Marunouchi T (1992) TNFα induces IL-6 production by astrocytes but not by microglia. *Brain Res* 583: 296–299

49   Sebire G, Emilie D, Wallon C, Hery C, Devergne O, Delfraissy JF, Galanaud P, Tardieu M (1993) In vitro production of IL-6, IL-1β, and tumor necrosis factor-α by human embryonic microglial and neural cells. *J Immunol* 150: 1517–1523

50   Sanna PP, Weiss F, Samson ME, Bloom FE, Pich EM (1995) Rapid induction of tumor necrosis factor a in the cerebrospinal fluid after intracerebroventricular injection of lipopolysaccharide revealed by a sensitive capture immuno-PCR assay. *Proc Natl Acad Sci USA* 92: 272–275

51   Navarra P, Pozzoli G, Brunetti L, Ragazzoni E, Besser M, Grossman A (1992) Interleukin-1β and interleukin-6 specifically increase the release of prostaglandin E_2 from rat hypothalamic explants *in vitro*. *Neuroendocrinology* 56: 61–68

52   Dinarello CA, Cannon JG, Wolff SM, Bernheim HA, Beutler B, Cerami A, Figari IS, Pal-

ladine Jr MA, O'Connor JV (1986) Tumor necrosis factor (cachectin) is an endogenous pyrogen and induces production of interleukin 1. *J Exp Med* 163: 1433–1450

53   Blalock JE, Smith EM (1981) Human leukocytic interferon (HuIFN-α): potent endorphin-like opioid activity. *Biochem Biophys Res Commun* 101: 472–478

54   Nakashima T, Murakami T, Murai Y, Hori T, Miyata S, Kiyohara T (1995) Naloxone suppresses the rising phase of fever induced by interferon-α. *Brain Res Bull* 37: 61–66

55   Nakashima T, Hori T, Kuriyama K, Matsuda T (1988) Effects of interferon-α on the activity of preoptic thermosensitive neurons in tissue slices. *Brain Res* 454: 361–367

56   Menzies RA, Patel R, Hall NRS, O'Grady MP, Rier SE (1992) Human recombinant interferon alpha inhibits naloxone binding to rat brain membranes. *Life Sci* 50: 227–232

57   Katsuura G, Arimura A, Koves K, Gottschall PE (1990) Involvement of organum vasculosum lamina terminalis and preoptic area in interleukin-1β-induced ACTH release. *Am J Physiol* 258: E163–E171

58   Matsumura K, Watanabe Y, Imai-Matsumura K, Connoly M, Koyama Y, Onoe H, Watanabe Y (1992) Mapping of prostaglandin E$_2$ binding sites in rat brain using quantitative autoradiography. *Brain Res* 581: 292–298

59   Watanabe Y, Watanabe Y, Hayaishi O (1988) Quantitative autoradiographic localization of prostaglandin E$_2$ binding sites in monkey diencephalon. *J Neurosci* 8: 2003–2010

60   Sugimoto Y, Shigemoto R, Namba T, Negishi M, Mizuno N, Narumiya S, Ichikawa A (1994) Distribution of the messenger RNA for the prostaglandin E receptor subtype EP$_3$ in the mouse nervous system. *Neuroscience* 62: 919–928

61   Matsuda T, Hori T, Nakashima T (1992) Thermal and PGE$_2$ sensitivity of the organum vasculosum lamina terminalis region and preoptic area in rat brain slices. *J Physiol (Lond)* 454: 197–212

62   Oka T, Aou S, Hori T (1994) Intracerebroventricular injection of prostaglandin E$_2$ induces thermal hyperalgesia in rats: the possible involvement of EP$_3$ receptors. *Brain Res* 663: 287–292

63   Oka T, Hosoi M, Oka K, Hori T (1997) Biphasic alteration in the trigeminal nociceptive neuronal responses after intracerebroventricular injection of prostaglandin E$_2$ in rats. *Brain Res* 749: 354–357

64   Coleman RA, Smith WL, Narumiya S (1994) VIII. International union of pharmacology classification of prostanoid receptors: properties, distribution and structure of the receptors and their subtypes. *Pharmacol Rev* 46: 205–229

65   Ushikubi F, Hirata M, Narumiya S (1995) Molecular biology of prostanoid receptors; an overview. *J Lipid Mediators Cell Signaling* 12: 343–359

66   Oka T, Hori T, Hosoi M, Oka K, Abe M, Kubo C (1997) Biphasic modulation in the trigeminal nociceptive neuronal responses by the intracerebroventricular prostaglandin E$_2$ may be mediated through different EP receptors subtypes in rats. *Brain Res* 771: 278–284

67   Hosoi M, Oka T, Hori T (1997) Prostaglandin E receptor EP$_3$ subtype is involved in thermal hyperalgesia through its actions in the preoptic hypothalamus and the diagonal

band of Broca in rats. *Pain* 71: 303–311

68   Honda A, Sugimoto Y, Namba T, Watabe A, Irie A, Negishi M, Narumiya S, Ichikawa A (1993) Cloning and expression of a cDNA for mouse prostaglandin E receptor EP_2 subtype. *J Biol Chem* 268: 7759–7762

69   Negishi M, Sugimoto Y, Irie A, Narumiya S, Ichikawa A (1993) Two isoforms of prostaglandin receptor EP_3 subtype. *J Biol Chem* 268: 9517–9521

70   Oka T, Hori T (1994) EP_1 receptor mediation of prostaglandin E_2-induced hyperthermia in rats. *Am J Physiol* 267: R289–R294

71   Oka K, Oka T, Hori T (1997) Prostaglandin E2 may induce hyperthermia through EP_1 receptor in the anterior wall of the third ventricle and neighboring preoptic regions. *Brain Res* 767: 92–99

72   Ando T, Ichijo T, Katafuchi T, Hori T (1995) Intracerebroventricular injection of prostaglandin E_2 increases splenic sympathetic nerve activity in rats. *Am J Physiol* 269: R662–R668

73   Oka T, Oka K, Hosoi M, Hori T (1996) Inhibition of peripheral interleukin-1β-induced hyperalgesia by the intracerebroventricular administration of diclofenac and α-melanocyte-stimulating hormone. *Brain Res* 736: 237–242

74   Maier SF, Wiertelak EP, Martin D, Watkins LR (1993) Interleukin-1 mediates the behavioral hyperalgesia produced by lithium chloride and endotoxin. *Brain Res* 623: 321–324

75   Laye S, Bluthe RM, Kent S, Combe C, Medina C, Parnet P, Kelley K, Dantzer R (1995) Subdiaphragmatic vagotomy blocks induction of IL-1β mRNA in mice brain in response to peripheral LPS. *Am J Physiol* 268: R1327–R1331

76   Masumura K, Cao C, Watanabe Y (1997) Possible role of cyclooxygenase-2 in the brain vasculature in febrile response. *Ann NY Acad Sci* 813: 302–306

77   Bernheim HA, Gilbert TM, Stitt JT (1980) Prostaglandin E levels in third ventricular cerebrospinal fluid of rabbit during fever and changes in body temperature. *J Physiol* (Lond) 301: 69–78

78   Poddubiuk ZM (1976) A comparison of the central actions of prostaglandins A_1, E_1, E_2, $F_{1\alpha}$ and $F_{2\alpha}$ in the rat. I. behavioral, antinociceptive and anticonvulsant actions of intraventricular prostaglandins in the rat. *Psychopharmacology* 50: 89–94

79   Ohkubo T, Shibata M, Takahashi H, Inoki R (1983) Effect of prostaglandin D_2 on pain and inflammation. *Jpn J Pharmacol* 33: 264–266

80   Bhattacharya SK (1986) The antinociceptive effect of intracerebroventricularly administered prostaglandin D_2 in the rat. *Psychopharmacology* 89: 121–124

81   Hori T, Oka T, Hosoi M, Aou S (1998) Pain modulatory actions of cytokines and prostaglandin E_2 in the brain. *Ann NY Acad Sci* 840: 269–281

Interleukin-1 and tumor necrosis factor: Rheumatoid arthritis and pain

David Martin

Department of Pharmacology, Amgen Inc., One Amgen Center Drive, Thousand Oaks, CA 91320, USA

Rheumatoid arthritis

Rheumatoid arthritis (RA) is a chronic inflammatory disorder of unknown etiology. It is a common disease, with a prevalence of 1 to 2% in the United States. Women are more commonly affected than men (average ratio is 3:1), and the disease produces substantial morbidity as well as an increase in mortality [1]. Although the etiology of RA is unknown, it is generally agreed that it represents an autoimmune disease that involves both the humoral and cellular arms of the immune response. A complex interaction of genetic, immunological, and local factors has been invoked to account for the differing patterns of joint involvement and progression of disease. Certainly RA may be caused by inflammatory CD4 T cells specific for a joint antigen which triggers the release of cytokines (and other mediators) that initiate local inflammation within the joint. This causes swelling, accumulation of polymorphonuclear leukocytes and macrophages, and damage to cartilage, leading to the destruction of the joint. Laboratory and clinical evidence suggests that proinflammatory cytokines, particularly interleukin-1 (IL-1) and tumor necrosis factor (TNF), have an important role in the pathogenesis of RA [2].

Besides the degenerative processes that occur at bone joints, due to the inflammatory processes, patients with RA suffer from pain which is not satisfactorily controlled with current therapies. This chapter will discuss the role of cytokines in the pathology of RA, cytokines and pain, and the clinical use of two cytokine inhibitors in RA and their effects on pain.

RA pathology

RA is characterized by a symmetrical and destructive polyarthritis affecting small and large synovial joints with associated systemic disturbances. In contrast to the acellular nature of normal synovial fluid, RA synovial fluid is enriched predominantly with neutrophils, but macrophages, T lymphocytes, and dendritic cells are also present. The increase in cellularity, however, is most obvious in the synovial membrane, which becomes infiltrated by cells recruited from the blood. The lining layer of the joint is increased from a couple of cells to 6–8 cells thick, and is comprised mostly of activated macrophages with an underlying layer of fibroblast-like cells. Neovascularization is prominent and there are many activated endothelial cells. The most abundant cells in the synovial membrane are macrophages and T lymphocytes, but plasma cells, dendritic cells, and activated fibroblasts are also found. Many of these cells are activated and express abundant human leukocyte antigen (HLA) class II and adhesion molecules of relevance in antigen presentation [3–8].

The major site of irreversible tissue damage originates at the junction of the synovium lining the joint capsule with the cartilage and bone, a region often termed the pannus, an area rich in macrophages. The cells of the pannus migrate over the underlying cartilage and into the subchondral bone, causing the subsequent erosion of these tissues [9]. The destruction of the cartilage seen in rheumatic disease is now considered to be mostly due to the activity of matrix metalloproteinases (MMPs), enzymes produced by activated macrophages and fibroblasts in response to proinflammatory cytokines, e.g. IL-1 and TNFα [10]. Furthermore, anti-inflammatory cytokines are also found in the RA joint such as IL-10, transforming growth factor β and interleukin-1 receptor antagonist (IL-1ra). These anti-inflammatory cytokines not only inhibit the production of proinflammatory cytokines but also indirectly downregulate other mediators involved in the destructive processes involved in the RA joint [11, 12].

IL-1 expression in animal models of RA

Studies in animal models of arthritis have further substantiated a proinflammatory role for IL-1. The mild and transient inflammation induced in rats by a single intraarticular injection of IL-1 became a more acute and destructive arthritis after multiple injections [13]. In a similar manner, injections of IL-1 markedly worsened the acute inflammation induced by the intraarticular administration of methylated bovine serum albumin into knees of non-sensitized mice [14]. In other studies, the chronic phase of antigen-induced arthritis in mice was reactivated by systemic or local injection of IL-1 [15], the onset and progression of spontaneous arthritis in MRL-*lpr* mice was enhanced by systemic infusion of IL-1 [16], and IL-1 injections promoted the development of collagen-induced arthritis only in mouse strains that were genetically susceptible to the disease [17]. The ability of IL-1 to stimulate both myelomonocytic cells and mesenchymal cells *in vitro* suggests that it plays a role both in chronic synovitis and in the tissue damage found in cartilage and bone [18, 19]. This was confirmed when IL-1 was injected into the knee joints of rabbits and was shown to induce acute arthritis with an accumulation of large numbers of leukocytes within the synovial lining and joint space and the loss of proteoglycan from articular cartilage [20–22]. These studies suggest that in human RA, IL-1 may be involved in induction of the acute phase, but may also contribute to the synovial inflammation.

Additional evidence for the importance of IL-1 in inflammatory arthritis is derived from studies on inhibition of cytokines. Neutralizing antibodies against murine IL-1 suppressed proteoglycan degradation, maintained normal proteoglycan synthesis and prevented both inflammation and cartilage destruction in antigen induced arthritis in mice [23, 24]. In addition, antibodies to IL-1 blocked the ability of media from cultured rheumatoid synovial tissue to degrade bovine cartilage *in vitro* [25]. The appearance of IL-1 in mammalian tissues during inflammation is accompanied by the endogenous IL-1 competitive antagonist IL-1ra, a protein without intrinsic activity. IL-1ra has high affinity for membrane IL-1 receptor, but due to the capacity of IL-1 to activate cells at very low receptor occupancy, a considerable molar excess of IL-1ra is required to inhibit IL-1 [26, 27]. IL-1ra also blocks the effects of IL-1 in diverse *in vitro* and *in vivo* models of joint destruction. IL-1ra inhibited IL-1-induced prostaglandin E_2 (PGE_2) and collagenase production by cultured rheumatoid synovial cells [28,29], PGE_2 production and bone resorption in cultured mouse and rat bones [30], and alterations in proteoglycan metabolism in explants of cultured human cartilage [31]. IL-1ra also attenuated the inflammatory effects of IL-1 and tissue destruction in various animal models, including streptococcal cell wall-induced arthritis in rats [32], lipopolysaccharide (LPS)-induced arthritis in rabbits [33], and collagen-induced arthritis in mice [34]. In addition, IL-1ra is effective in inhibiting the synovitis and cartilage proteoglycan loss caused by intra-articular injection of IL-1 [35]. Furthermore, evaluation of IL-1ra in an established antigen-induced arthritis showed a potent antifibrotic activity in rabbits [36]. However, other related studies indicated that IL-1ra had no inhibitory effect on swelling, leukocyte accumulation or cartilage proteoglycan loss when administered to rabbits with acute antigen-induced arthritis [37]. Overall, these studies suggest that various *in vitro* and *in vivo* models of arthritis offer evidence for the importance of IL-1 as a mediator of both acute and chronic pathophysiological events.

IL-1 and human RA

The use of peripheral blood cells, synovial fluid cells, synovial fluid itself and synovial tissue from patients with RA further substantiate the conclusion that IL-1 is produced in increased amounts in this disease. Peripheral blood monocytes from RA patients produced more IL-1 *in vitro* in comparison with cells from normal subjects [38]. Similarly, monocytes from rheumatoid synovial fluids produced more IL-1 after *in vitro* stimulation than did peripheral blood cells from the same patients [39]. Furthermore, synovial fluid IL-1 levels were correlated with some clinical and histological parameters of disease activity in patients with RA [40].

The expression of IL-1ra mRNA is upregulated in RA joints as is the protein in RA synovial fluid and cell cultures [41, 42]. The localization of IL-1ra is to CD68 macrophages [41]. Normal joint tissues express very little IL-1ra but expression increases in RA patients. IL-1ra was found in high concentrations in synovial fluids of patients with RA when compared to patients with infectious or non-rheumatoid inflammatory arthritis [43]. The synovial fluid IL-1ra levels correlated with concentrations of neutrophils in these fluids and may represent production primarily by these cells. Elevated levels of synovial fluid IL-1ra, in comparison with IL-1, were correlated with a more rapid resolution of acute knee arthritis in patients with Lyme disease [44]. These observations suggest that endogenously produced IL-1ra present in synovial fluid may penetrate the synovial tissue and inhibit local inflammation. Furthermore, soluble IL-1 receptor (sIL-1R) has been detected in RA tissues, initially in synovial fluid [45]. This was first found as an IL-1β binding protein and was subsequently identified using monoclonal antibody as the type II IL-1R. This receptor is not involved in signaling and appears to function not only as a decoy on the cell surface, but also as an inhibitor since it binds proIL-1β, mature IL-1β, but not IL-1ra [46].

The available evidence therefore suggests that the accumulation of leukocytes and loss of proteoglycan from articular cartilage in inflammatory joint diseases may be due to the direct or indirect action of IL-1. Inhibition of biological action of IL-1 or inhibition of its synthesis would therefore be a possible therapeutic mode of intervention.

RA and pain

The pattern of symptoms in RA is complex and includes pain and tenderness not only in joints that are directly involved with the disease process but also in surrounding, apparently normal tissues. Referred pain syndromes may also occur. The magnitude of symptoms may not necessarily correlate with the severity of the underlying disease and symptoms may persist even when disease exacerbations have apparently settled.

Neurophysiological mechanisms underlying pain in RA remain unclear. Experimental models of inflammatory arthritis suggest that changes of neuronal sensitivity at both peripheral and central levels may be important [47]. Within the joint, injury or inflammation inevitably produces sensitization and subsequent activation of articulator sensory receptors [48]. Although peripheral sensitization is widely held to be responsible for pain and tenderness over inflamed or damaged joints, it does not necessarily account for other symptoms observed in RA. Sensitization of neurons in the dorsal horn of the spinal cord has also been reported under experimental conditions [49, 50], but while this has been postulated to influence pain sensation during arthritis, direct evidence from clinical situations is lacking. Furthermore, capsaicin which produces pain, vasodilatation, hyperalgesia and allodynia was used to explore sensory mechanisms in both normal and RA patients [51]. Such studies are used to quantify cutaneous axon-reflex responses as an indirect marker of peripheral sensory activity. In degenerative arthritis of the spine, capsaicin-induced skin flares were reduced [52], whereas selective increases over inflamed joints were apparent in RA. At other reference sites, away from inflamed RA joints, skin flares were similar to those observed in normal controls [53]. The conclusion from this latter study was that, while a selective increase of peripheral sensory fibre activity was apparent over joints involved in RA, a generalized upregulation was not apparent and was therefore unlikely to be contributing to more general symptoms in this disorder [53].

IL-1 and pain

Normal cartilage cells can produce a wide spectrum of cytokines including IL-1, TNFα, and IL-6 [54]. Cytokines such as IL-1 and TNF mediate pain, hyperalgesia and allodynia [55]. The evidence for IL-1 as a mediator of pain is as follows.

Interleukin-1 has been shown to have nociceptive actions found during *in vivo* and *in vitro* models of pain and hyperalgesia. IL-1β is produced by activated macrophages and a large variety of other cell types including B-lymphocytes and endothelial cells and upon administration causes hyperalgesia [56–58]. It is interesting to note that IL-1α appears not to have hyperalgesic actions [59].

Initial studies demonstrated mechanical hyperalgesia with intraplantar injections of IL-1β in the rat. Subsequently, there have been several reports of IL-1β-induced mechanical and thermal hyperalgesia. Intraperitoneal injections of LPS or IL-1β (µg/kg range) or local administration of IL-1β (pg) have been shown to induce mechanical and thermal hyperalgesia in the rat [56, 60]. Furthermore, studies have demonstrated that intraplantar injection of IL-1β can induce hyperalgesia not only in the injected paw but also in the contralateral paw [58, 59]. However, the bilateral hyperalgesia is still equivocal since other investigators have not been able to duplicate these studies [61]. Presently there is no explanation for these discrepancies, however, it is possible that procedural differences could explain the differences for the actions of IL-1β.

Cytokines in general appear to be involved in either the local or global hyperalgesia that occurs in inflammatory disorders. IL-1β appears to be a component of inflammatory pain, and studies demonstrating that IL-1β mediates hyperalgesia when injected into either the paw or knee joint support the above statement. However, it is not clear whether IL-1β acts directly on the nociceptive neuron to cause sensitization or activation, or whether its actions are indirect via the release of secondary mediators such as kinins or prostaglandins [62].

Electrophysiological studies have shown that IL-1β injected into the hind paw or knee joint increased the spontaneous firing of sensory nerves [63]. Furthermore, IL-1β increased neuronal responses to noxious heat and cold stimuli and decreased the threshold for firing to pressure stimulation [63]. In addition, it has been shown that joint mechanonociceptors respond to IL-1β with a sustained increase in activity [64]. As mentioned before, most of these effects could be mediated indirectly. However, a recent study demonstrated in dissociated dorsal root ganglion cells of rat, that IL-1β causes an immediate increase in intracellular concentration of Ca^{2+} ions, suggesting that IL-1β may be acting directly on the sensory neurons [65].

Hyperalgesia and IL-1ra

Further support for IL-1β in the mediation of hyperalgesia comes from the use of IL-1ra. Systemic administration of IL-1ra was shown to inhibit hyperalgesia mediated by LPS, lithium chloride, CFA, or IL-1 [56, 60, 66]. Furthermore, Watkins et al. demonstrated that LPS-induced hyperalgesia was not attenuated by the cyclo-oxygenase inhibitor indomethacin [56]. However, indomethacin has been shown to block IL-1β responses in other studies. Thus the involvement of prostaglandins in the behavioral hyperalgesia seen with IL-1β appears equivocal.

In general, the majority of studies have shown that exogenously injected IL-1β is pro-nociceptive in animals but do not clearly address the question as to whether IL-1β has a role in pain perception in man. This question can only be answered when an IL-1 receptor antagonist is used clinically, but the animal studies do suggest that IL-1 may be an important pain mediator in humans.

The interleukin-1 receptor antagonist was recently evaluated in a placebo controlled double blind clinical trial over a 24 week period in RA patients. Patients that received IL-1ra demonstrated a significant reduction in tender joint scores and associated pain when compared to placebo treated patients. Furthermore, IL-1ra treatment was associated with a significant improvement in the physician and patient's assessment when compared to the placebo group [67]. The attenuation in pain and number of tender joints is consistent with IL-1ra inhibiting IL-1-mediated pain. However, the reduction in pain and tender joints could also be due to an inhibition of the local inflammation. Therefore, further IL-1ra studies are required to dissect out whether IL-1ra attenuates pain directly and/or by inhibiting the local inflammation.

TNF and RA

TNF appears to have a role in the pathogenesis of RA [2, 68]. TNF has been found to induce the release of matrix metalloproteases from neutrophils, fibroblasts, and chondrocytes [69–71], induces the expression of endothelial adhesion molecules involved in the migration of leukocytes to extravascular sites of inflammation [72], and stimulates the release of other proinflammatory cytokines [73, 74]. TNF concentrations are increased in the synovial fluid of persons with active RA [75, 76], and increased plasma levels of TNF are associated with joint pain [77]. Furthermore, administration of TNF antagonists to patients with RA has been shown to reduce symptoms [78–80].

There are two distinct cell surface TNF receptors, designated p55 and p75 [81, 82]. Soluble, truncated versions of membrane TNFs, consisting of only the extracellular, ligand-binding domain, are present in body fluids and are thought to be involved in regulating TNF activity [83, 84]. Soluble tumor necrosis factor receptors (sTNFR) have been detected in synovial tissue and at the junction between cartilage and pannus [85, 86]. Their levels are increased in serum and synovial fluid in RA and in other autoimmune and inflammatory conditions.

TNF and hyperalgesia

Most of the experimental evidence linking TNF-alpha in hyperalgesia is from behavioral models of hyperalgesia. Behavioral hyperalgesia has been demonstrated after local administration of TNFα into rat paws and following systemic administration using a tail flick hyperalgesia model [57, 87, 88]. Local administration of TNFα mediated an indomethacin sensitive hyperalgesia which was antagonized by antisera to IL-1β [89]. The hyperalgesia mediated by TNFα when administered locally could be attenuated by IL-1 antagonists and indomethacin. The block by these agents was incomplete, and there seemed to be a sympathetic component to TNF-induced hyperalgesia [89]. Thus the local effects of TNF seem to involve some endogenous production of IL-1. It was also noted that IL-1-induced hyperalgesia was not sensitive to TNF antisera.

Administration of TNFα intraperitoneally induced hyperalgesia as observed in the tail flick test and was attenuated by subdiaphragmatic vagotomy, suggesting a neural mode of action. In addition, IL-1ra attenuated the TNFα-mediated hyperalgesia, suggesting that endogenous IL-1β was an active component of the hyperalgesic response [87].

A series of human clinical trials evaluating TNF inhibitors in RA have demonstrated beneficial effects on a number of end points relating to pain. An example is the soluble TNF receptor (p75) linked to the Fc portion of human IgG1 (TNF:Fc) [80]. In this phase three trial, TNF:Fc produced significant improvement in all measures of disease activity. A clear dose-response relation was observed in the numbers of swollen or tender joints, and patients who received the highest dose (16 mg per square meter of body surface area) of TNF:Fc had the greatest improvement (Fig. 1). The 16 mg dose of TNFR:Fc was associated with the great-

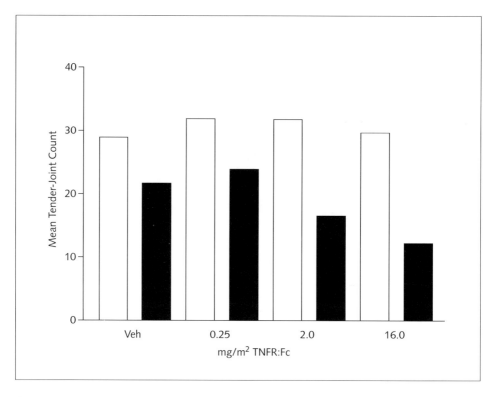

Figure 1
Effect of three months treatment with TNFR:Fc in rheumatoid arthritis patients on mean ten-
der joint counts. The clear columns represent baseline measurements (before treatment
starts), and the shaded columns represent treatment groups (three months later). TNFR:Fc
significantly (p < 0.001) reduced the number of tender joints over the course of the treat-
ment. The P values were obtained from the analysis of variance comparing all four treatment
groups in terms of percent change from base line to three months with a model that con-
tained main effects of treatment and center (see [80] for details). Data taken from [80].

est reduction in the number of swollen or tender joints and the difference was
apparent by the end of week two and was most pronounced at the end of treatment (at three months). Similarly, significant reductions in pain (Fig. 2) and duration of morning stiffness, improvement in the quality of life and both physician
and patient global assessments were observed [80]. However, since TNF:Fc, like
other TNF inhibitors, cause a general reduction in all signs of arthritis, including
joint swelling, the reduction in pain could have been due to the anti-inflammato-

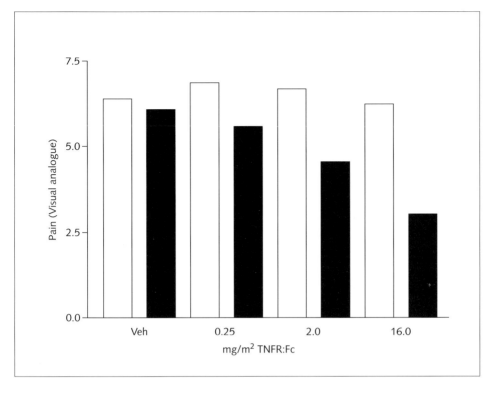

Figure 2
Effect of three months treatment with TNFR:Fc in rheumatoid arthritis patients on pain (a visual-analogue scale from 0 (no pain) to 10 (severe pain). The clear columns represent baseline measurements (before treatment starts), and the shaded columns represent treatment groups (three months later). TNFR:Fc significantly (p = 0.001) reduced pain over the course of the treatment. The P values were obtained from the analysis of variance comparing all four treatment groups in terms of percent change from base line to three months with a model that contained main effects of treatment and center (see [80] for details). Data taken from [80].

ry effects of these inhibitors by reducing the presence of other mediators of hyperalgesia in the joint.

In addition, based on preclinical and clinical data, it is suggested that cytokines may be fruitful as targets for novel analgesic drugs for such conditions as phantom limb pain, reflex sympathetic dystrophy, traumatic nerve injuries, herpes zoster virus, trigeminal neuralgia and diabetic neuropathy which are presently not adequately managed.

References

1   Linos A, Worthington JW, O'Fallon WM, Kurland LT (1980) The epidemiology of rheumatoid arthritis in Rochester, Minnesota: A study of incidence, prevalence and mortality. *Am J Epidemiol* 111: 87–98

2   Arend WP, Dayer JM (1995) Inhibition of the production and effects of interleukin-1 and tumor necrosis factor alpha in rheumatoid arthritis. *Arthritis Rheum* 38: 151–160

3   Cush JJ, Lipsky PE (1988) Phenotypic analysis of synovial tissue and peripheral blood lymphocytes isolated from patients with rheumatoid arthritis. *Arthritis Rheum* 31: 1230–1238

4   Johnson BA, Haines GK, Harlow LA, Koch AE (1993) Adhesion molecule expression in human synovial tissue. *Arthritis Rheum* 36: 137–146

5   Janossy G, Panayi G, Duke O, Bofill M, Poulter LW, Goldstein G (1981) Rheumatoid arthritis: a disease of T-lymphocyte/macrophage immunoregulation. *Lancet* ii 839–841

6   Klareskog L, Forsum, U, Scheynius A, Kabelitz, D, Wigzell H (1982) Evidence in support of a self perpetuating HLA-DR dependent delayed type cell reaction in rheumatoid arthritis. *Proc Natl Acad Sci USA* 72: 3632–3636

7   Morales-Ducret J, Wayner E, Elices MJ, Alvaro-Garcia JM, Zvaifler NJ, Firestein GS (1992) Alpha 4/beta 1 integrin (VLA-4) ligands in arthritis: I. Vascular cell adhesion molecule 1 expression in synovium and on fibroblast-like synoviocytes. *J Immunol* 149: 1424–1451

8   Helmer ME, Glass, D, Coblyn JS, Jacobson JG (1986) Very late activation antigens on rheumatoid synovial fluid T lymphocytes: association with stages of T cell activation. *J Clin Invest* 78: 696–702

9   Allard SA, Muirden KD, Camplejohn KL, Maini RN (1987) Chondrocyte derived cells and matrix at the rheumatoid cartilage-pannus junction identified with monoclonal antibodies. *Rheumatol Int* 7: 153–159

10 Vincenti MP, Clark IM, Brinckerhoff CE (1994) Using inhibitors of metalloproteinases to treat arthritis. *Arthritis Rheum* 37: 1115–1126

11 Wright JK, Cawston TE, Hazelman BL (1991) Transforming growth factor beta stimulates the production of the tissue inhibitor of metalloproteinases (TIMP) by human synovial and skin fibroblasts. *Biochem Biophys Acta* 1094: 207–210.

12 Feldmann M, Brennan FM, Maini RN (1996) Role of cytokines in rheumatoid arthritis. *Annu Rev Immunol* 14: 397–440

13 Chandrasekhar S, Harvey AK, Hrubey PS, Bendele AM (1990) Arthritis induced by interleukin-1 is dependent on the site and frequency of intraarticular injection. *Clin Immunol Immunopathol* 55: 382–400

14 Staite ND, Richard KA, Aspar DG, Franz KA, Galinet LA, Dunn CJ (1990) Induction of acute erosive monarticular arthritis in mice by interleukin-1 and methylated bovine serum albumin. *Arthritis Rheum* 33: 253–260

15 Van de Loo AAJ, Arntz OJ, van den Berg WB (1992) Flare-up of experimental arthritis in mice with murine recombinant IL-1. *Clin Exp Immunol* 87: 196–202

16   Hom JT, Cole H, Bendele AM (1990) Interleukin-1 enhances the development of spontaneous arthritis in MRL/Ipr mice. *Clin Immunol Immunopathol* 55: 109–119

17   Hom JT, Cole H., Estridge T, Gliszczynski VL (1992) Interleukin-1 enhances the development of type II collagen-induced arthritis only in susceptible and not in resistant mice. *Clin Immunol Immunopathol* 62: 56–65

18   Henderson B, Pettipher ER, Higgs GA (1987) Mediators of rheumatoid arthritis. *Br Med Bull* 43: 415–428

19   Duff G (1989) Interleukin-1 in inflammatory joint disease. In: Bomford R, Henderson B (eds): *Interleukin-1 inflammation and disease.* Elsevier, Amsterdam, 243–255

20   Pettipher ER, Higgs GA, Henderson B (1986) Interleukin-1 induces leukocyte infiltration and cartilage proteoglycan degradation in the synovial joint. *Proc Natl Acad Sci USA* 83: 8749–8753

21   Henderson B, Pettipher ER (1988) Comparison of the *in vivo* inflammatory activities after intra-articular injection of natural and recombinant IL-1α and IL-1β in the rabbit. *Biochem Pharmacol* 37: 4171–4176

22   Feige U, Karbowski A, Rordorf-Adam C, Pataki A (1989) Arthritis induced by continuous infusion of hr-interleukin-1α into the rabbit knee-joint. *Int J Tiss Reac* XI: 225–238

23   Fons, AF, van de Loo FA, Onno J, Arntz, Otterness IG, van den Berg WB (1992) Protection against cartilage proteoglycan synthesis inhibition by antiinterleukin-1 antibodies in experimental arthritis. *J Rheumatol* 19: 348–356.

24   Van den Berg WB, Joostens LAB, Helsen M, van de Loo FA (1994) Amelioration of established murine collagen-induced arthritis with anti-IL-1 treatment. *Clin Exp Immunol* 95: 237–243

25   Chu CQ, Field M, Feldman M, Maini RN (1991) Localization of tumor necrosis factor alpha in synovial tissues and at the cartilage-pannus junction in patients with rheumatoid arthritis. *Arthritis Rheum* 34: 1125–1132

26   Dripps DJ, Brandhuber BJ, Thompson RC, Eisenberg SP (1991) Interleukin-1 (IL-1) receptor antagonist binds to the 80-kDa IL-1 receptor but does not initiate signal transduction. *J Biol Chem* 266: 1331–1334

27   Dripps DJ, Verderber E, Ng RC, Thompson RC, Eisenberg, SP (1991) Interleukin-1 receptor antagonist binds to the type II interleukin-1 receptor on B cells and neutrophils. *J Biol Chem* 226: 20311–20315

28   Arend WP, Welgus HG, Thompson RC, Eisenberg SP (1990) Biological properties of recombinant human monocyte-derived interleukin-1 receptor antagonist. *J Clin Invest* 85: 1694–1697

29   Seckinger P, Kaufmann M-T, Dayer J-M (1990) An interleukin-1 inhibitor affects both cell-associated interleukin-1-induced T cell proliferation and PGE_2/collagenase production by human dermal fibroblasts and synovial cells. *Immunobiology* 180: 316–327

30   Seckinger P, Klein-Nulend J, Alander C, Thompson RC, Dayer J-M, Raisz LG (1990) Natural and recombinant human IL-1 receptor antagonists block the effects of IL-1 on bone resorpotion and prostaglandin production. *J Immunol* 145: 4181–4184

31   Seckinger P, Yaron I, Meyer FA, Yaron M, Dayer J-M (1990) Modulation of the effects of interleukin-1 on glycosaminoglycan synthesis by the urine-derived interleukin-1 inhibitor, but not by interleukin-6. *Arthritis Rheum* 33: 1807–1814

32   Schwab JH, Anderle SK, Brown RR, Dalldorf FG, Thompson RC (1991) Pro- and anti-inflammatory roles of interleukin-1 in recurrence of bacterial cell wall-induced arthritis in rats. *Infect Immun* 59: 4436–4442

33   Matsukawa A, Ohkawara S, Maeda T, Takagi K, Yoshinaga M (1993) Production of IL-1 and IL-1 receptor antagonist and the pathological significance in lipopolysaccharide-induced arthritis in rabbits. *Clin Exp Immunol* 93: 206–211

34   Wooley PH, Whalen JD, Chapman, DL, Berger AE, Richard KA, Aspar DG, Staite ND (1993) The effect of an interleukin-1 receptor antagonist protein on type II collagen-induced arthritis and antigen-induced arthritis in mice. *Arthritis Rheum* 36: 1305–1314

35   Henderson B, Thompson RC, Hardingham T, Lewthwaite J (1991) Inhibition of inter-leukin-1-induced synovitis and articular cartilage proteoglycan loss in the rabbit knee by recombinant human interleukin-1 receptor antagonist. *Cytokine* 3: 246–249

36   Lewthwaite J, Blake SM, Thompson RC, Hardingham TE, Henderson B (1995) Antifi-brotic action of interleukin-1 receptor antagonist in lipine monoarticular arthritis. *Annals Rheumat Diseases* 54: 591–596

37   Lewthwaite J, Blake SM, Hardingham TE, Warden PJ, Henderson B (1994) The effect of recombinant human interleukin 1 receptor antagonist on the induction phase of anti-gen induced arthritis in the rabbit. *J Rheumatol* 21: 467–472

38   Ruschen S, Stellberg W, Warnatz H (1992) Kinetics of cytokine secretion by mononu-clear cells of the blood from rheumatoid arthritis patients are different from those of healthy controls. *Clin Exp Immunol* 89: 32–37

39   Dularay B, Westacott CI, Elson CJ (1992) IL-1 secreting cell assay and its application to cells from patients with rheumatoid arthritis. *Br J Rheumatol* 31: 19–24

40   Holt I, Cooper RG, Denton J, Meager A, Hopkins SJ (1992) Cytokine inter-relation-ships and their association with disease activity in arthritis. *Br J Rheumatol* 31: 725–733

41   Firestein GS, Berger AE, Tracey DE, Chosay JG, Chapman DL, Paine MM, Yu C, Zvai-fler NJ (1992) IL-1 receptor antagonist protein production and gene expression in rheumatoid arthritis and osteoarthritis synovium. *J Immunol* 149: 1054–1062

42   Koch AE, Kunkel SL, Chensue SW, Haines GK, Strieter RM (1992) Expression of inter-leukin-1 and interleukin-1 receptor antagonist by human rheumatoid synovial tissue macrophages. *Clin Immunol Immunopathol* 65: 23–29

43   Malyak M, Swaney RE, Arend WP (1993) Levels of synovial fluid interleukin-1 recep-tor antagonist in rheumatoid arthritis and other arthropathies: potential contribution from synovial fluid neutrophils. *Arthritis Rheum* 36: 781–789

44   Miller LC, Lynch EA, Isa S, Logan JW, Dinarello CA, Steere AC (1993) Balance of syn-ovial fluid IL-1β and IL-1 receptor antagonist and recovery from Lyme disease. *Lancet* 341: 146–148

45   Symons, JA., Eastgate, JA., Duff, GW (1991) Purification and characterization of a novel soluble receptor for interleukin-1. *J Exp Med* 174: 1251–1254

216

46   Symons JA, Young PR, Duff GW (1995) Soluble type II interleukin 1 (IL-1) receptor binds and blocks processing of IL-1β precursor and loses affinity for IL-1 receptor antagonist. *Proc Natl Acad Sci USA* 92: 1714–1718

47   Schaible H, Grubb, BD (1993) Afferent and spinal mechanisms of joint pain. *Pain* 55: 554–557

48   Schaible H, Schmidt, RF (1988) Time course of mechanosensitivity changes in articular afferents during a developing experimental arthritis. *J Neurophysiol* 60: 2180–2195

49   Neugebauer V, Schaible H-G (1990) Evidence for a central component in the sensitisation of spinal neurones with joint input during development of acute arthritis in cat's knee. *J Neurophysiol* 64: 299–311

50   Dougherty PM, Sluka KA, Sorkin KN, Westlund KN, Willis WD (1992) Neural changes in acute arthritis in monkeys. I. Parallel enhancement of responses of spinothalmic tract neurones to mechanical stimulation and excitatory amino acids. *Brain Res Rev* 17: 1–13

51   Simone DA, Baumann TK, LaMotte RH (1989) Dose-dependent pain and mechanical hyperalgesia in humans after intradermal injection of capsaicin. *Pain* 38: 99–107

52   LeVasseur SA, Gibson SJ, Helme RD (1990) The measurement of capsaicin- sensitive sensory nerve fibre function in elderly patients with pain. *Pain* 41: 19–25

53   Jolliffe VA, Anand P, Kidd BL (1995) Assessment of cutaneous sensory and autonomic axon reflexes in rheumatoid arthritis. *Ann Rheum Dis* 54: 251–255

54   Chu CQ, Field M, Allard S, Abney E, Feldman M, Maini, RN (1992) Detection of cytokines at the cartilage/pannus junction in patients with rheumatoid arthritis: implications for the role of cytokines in cartilage destruction and repair. *Br J Rheumatol* 31: 653–661

55   Watkins LR, Maier SF, Goehler LE (1995) Immune activation: the role of pro-inflammatory cytokines in inflammation, illness responses and pathological pain states. *Pain* 63: 289–302

56   Watkins LR, Wiertelak EP, Goehler LE, Smith KP, Martin D, Maier SF (1994) Characterization of cytokine-induced hyperalgesia. *Brain Res* 654: 15–26

57   Davis AJ, Perkins MN (1994) The involvement of bradykinin B1 and B2 receptor mechanisms in cytokine-induced mechanical hyperalgesia in the rat. *Br J Pharmacol* 113: 63–68

58   Perkins MN, Kelly D (1994) Interleukin-1β induced-desArg⁹bradykinin-mediated thermal hyperalgesia in the rat. *Neuropharmacology* 33: 657–660

59   Ferreira SH, Lorenzetti BB, Bristow AF, Poole, S (1988) Interleukin-1β as a potent hyperalgesic agent antagonized by a tripeptide analogue. *Nature* 334: 698–700

60   Maier SF, Wiertelak, EP, Martin D, and Watkins LR (1993) Interleukin-1 mediates the behavioral hyperalgesia produced by lithium chloride and endotoxin. *Brain Res* 623: 21–24

61   Follenfant RL, Nakamura CM, Henderson B, Higgs GA (1989) Inhibition by neuropeptides of interleukin-1β-induced, prostaglandin-independent hyperalgesia. *Br J Pharmacol* 98: 41–43

62   Scheweizer A, Feige U, Fontanna A, Muller K, Dinarello CA (1988) Interleukin-1

enhances pain reflexes. Mediation through increased prostaglandin E_2 levels. *Agents and Actions* 25: 246–251

63   Fukuota, H, Kawatani M, Hisamitsu T, Takeshige C (1994) Cutaneous hyperalgesia induced by peripheral injection of interleukin-1β in the rat. *Brain Res* 657: 133–140

64   Kelly DC, Ashgar AUR, McQueen DS (1996) Effects of bradykinin and desArg[9]-bradykinin on afferent neural discharge in interleukin-1beta-treated knee joints. *Br J Pharmacol* 117: 90P

65   Kawatani M, Birder L (1992) Interleukin-1 facilitates Ca^{2+} release in acutely dissociated dorsal root ganglion (DRG) cells of rat. *Neurosci Abst* 18: 691

66   Safieh-Garabedian B, Poole S, Allchorne A, Winter J, Woolf CJ (1995) Contribution of interleukin-1β to the inflammation-induced increase in nerve growth factor levels and inflammatory hyperalgesia. *Br J Pharmacol* 115: 1265–1275

67   Nuki G, Rozman, B, Pavelka, K, Emery P, Lockabaugh J, Musikic P (1997) Interleukin-1 receptor antagonist continues to demonstrate clinical improvement in rheumatoid arthritis. *Arthritis & Rheumatism* 40: 1159, S224

68   Brennan FM, Feldmann M (1992) Cytokines in autoimmunity. *Curr Opin Immunol* 4: 745–749.

69   Shingu M, Nagai Y, Isayama T, Naono T, Nobunaga M, Nagai Y (1993) The effects of cytokines on metalloproteinase inhibitors (TIMP) and collagenase production by human chondrocytes and TIMP production by synovial cells and endothelial cells. *Clin Exp Immunol* 94: 145–149

70   MacNaul KL, Chartrain N, Lark M, Tocci MJ, Hutchinson NI (1992) Differential effects of IL-1 and TNFα on the expression of stromelysin, collagenase and their natural inhibitor, TIMP, in rheumatoid human synovial fibroblasts. *Matrix Suppl* 1: 198–199

71   Ahmadzadeh N, Shingu M, Nobunaga M (1990) The effect of recombinant tumor necrosis factor-alpha on superoxide and metalloproteinase production by synovial cells and chondrocytes. *Clin Exp Rheumatol* 8: 387–391

72   Moser RB, Schleiffenbaum B, Groscurth P, Fehr J (1989) Interleukin 1 and tumor necrosis factor stimulate human vascular endothelial cells to promote transendothelial neutrophil passage. *J Clin Invest* 83: 444–455

73   Nawroth PP, Bank I, Handley D, Cassimeris J, Chess L, Stern D (1986) Tumor necrosis factor/cachectin interacts with endothelial cell receptors to induce release of interleukin 1. *J Exp Med* 163: 1363–1375.

74   Brennan FM, Chantry D, Jackson A, Maini R, Feldmann M (1989) Inhibitory effect of TNFα antibodies on synovial cell interleukin-1 production in rheumatoid arthritis. *Lancet* 2: 244–247

75   Yodlowski ML, Hubbard JR, Kispert J, Keller K, Sledge CB, Steinberg JJ (1990) Antibody to interleukin-1 inhibits the cartilage degradative and thymocyte proliferative actions of rheumatoid synovial culture medium. *J Rheumatol* 17: 1600–1607

76   Saxne T, Pallidino MA Jr, Heinegard D, Talal N, Wollheim FA (1988) Detection of tumor necrosis factor alpha but not tumor necrosis factor beta in rheumatoid arthritis synovial fluid and serum. *Arthritis Rheum* 31: 1041–1045

77   Beckham JC, Caldwell DS, Peterson BL (1992) Disease severity in rheumatoid arthritis: relationship of plasma tumor necrosis factor-alpha, soluble interleukin 2-receptor, soluble CD4/CD8 ratio, neopterin, and fibrin D-dimer to traditional severity and functional measures. *J Clin Immunol* 12; 353–361

78   Eillott MJ, Maini RN, Feldmann M (1994) Repeated therapy with monoclonal antibody to tumor necrosis factor alpha (cA2) in patients with rheumatoid arthritis. *Lancet* 344: 1125–1127

79   Rankin EC, Choy EHS, Kassimos D, Kingsley GH, Sopwith AM, Isenberg DA, Panayi GS (1995) The therapeutic effects of an engineered human anti-tumor necrosis factor alpha antibody (CDP571) in rheumatoid arthritis. *Br J Rheumatol* 34: 334–342

80   Moreland LW, Baumgartner SW, Schiff MH, Tindall EA, Fleischmann RM, Weaver AL, Ettlinger RE, Cohen S, Koopman WJ, Mohler K et al (1997) Treatment of rheumatoid arthritis with a recombinant human tumor necrosis factor receptor (p75)-Fc fusion protein. *N Engl J Med* 337: 141–147

81   Smith CA, Davis T, Anderson D (1990) A receptor for tumor necrosis factor defines an unusual family of cellular and viral proteins. *Science* 248: 1019–1023

82   Loetscher H, Pan YC, Lahm HW (1990) Molecular cloning and expression of the human 55 kd tumor necrosis factor receptor. *Cell* 61: 351–359

83   Engelmann H, Aderka D, Rubinstein M, Rotman D, Wallach D (1989) A tumor necrosis factor binding-protein purified to homogeneity from human urine protects cells from tumor necrosis factor toxicity. *J Biol Chem* 264: 11974–11980

84   Olsson I, Lantz M, Nilsson E (1989) Isolation and characterization of a tumor necrosis factor binding protein from urine. *Eur J Haematol* 42: 270–275

85   Deleuran BW, Chu CQ, Field M (1992) Localization of tumor necrosis factor receptors in the synovial tissue and cartilage-pannus junction in patients with rheumatoid arthritis; implications for local actions of tumor necrosis factor alpha. *Arthritis Rheum.* 35: 1170–1178

86   Westacott CI, Atkins RM, Dieppe PA, Elson CJ (1994) Tumor necrosis factor-alpha receptor expression on chondrocytes isolated from human articular cartilage. *J Rheumatol* 21: 1710–1715

87   Watkins LR, Goehler LE, Relton J, Brewer MT, Maier SF (1995) Mechanisms of TNF-induced hyperalgesia. *Brain Res* 692: 244–250

88   Woolf CA, Allchorne A, Safieh-Garabedian B, Poole S (1997) Cytokines, nerve growth factor and inflammatory hyperalgesia: the contribution of tumor necrosis factor alpha. *Brit J Pharmacol* 121: 417–424

89   Cunha FQ, Poole S, Lorenzetti BB, Ferreira SH (1992) The pivotal role of tumor necrosis factor alpha in the development of inflammatory hyperalgesia. *Brit J Pharmacol* 107: 660–664

Index

http://www.birkhauser.ch

Check our Highlights for new and notable titles selected monthly
in each field

PIR
Progress in Inflammation Research

Medicinal Fatty Acids in Inflammation

Kremer, J.M.,
Albany Medical College, Albany, USA (Ed.)

This volume is a unique assembly of contributions focusing
on the biochemical, immunological and clinical benefits of
n-3 fatty acids in inflammation.

Leading clinical investigators from fields as diverse as
rheumatology, dermatology, nephrology, gastroenterology
and neurology have authored chapters. The basic scientific
underpinnings of their findings are elucidated as well.

The work is a highly accessible, one-of-a-kind source
which will well serve lipid researchers, graduate students,
dieticians and members of the food industry.

Contents

List of contributors

Preface

Calder, P. C.:
n-3 Polyunsaturated fatty acids and mononuclear
phagocyte function

Zurier, R. B.:
Gammalinolenic acid treatment of rheumatoid arthritis

Ziboh, V. A.:
The role of n-3 fatty acids in psoriasis

Horrobin, D. F.:
n-6 Fatty acids and nervous system diorders

Fernandes, G.:
n-3 Fatty acids on autoimmune disease and apoptosis

Belluzzi, A. and Miglio, F.:
n-3 Fatty acids in the treatment of Crohn's disease

Rodgers, J. B.:
n-3 Fatty acids in the treatment of ulcerative colitis

Geusens, P. P.:
n-3 Fatty acids in the treatment of rheumatoid arthritis

Grande, J. P. and Donadio, J. V.:
n-3 Polyunsaturated fatty acids in the treatment of
patients with IgA nephropathy

Subject index

PIR – Progress in Inflammation Research
Kremer, J.M. (Ed.)
Medicinal Fatty Acids in Inflammation
1998. 154 pages. Hardcover
ISBN 3-7643-5854-8

BioSciences with Birkhäuser

(Prices are subject to change without notice. 10/98)

For orders originating from all over the world
except USA and Canada:

Birkhäuser Verlag AG
P.O. Box 133
CH-4010 Basel / Switzerland
Fax: +41 / 61 / 205 07 92
e-mail: orders@birkhauser.ch

For orders originating in the USA and
Canada:

Birkhäuser Boston, Inc.
333 Meadowland Parkway
USA-Secaucus, NJ 07094-2491
Fax: +1 / 201 348 4033
e-mail: orders@birkhauser.com

Birkhäuser

PIR
Progress in Inflammation Research

Inducible Enzymes in the Inflammatory Response

Willoughby, D. A., Tomlinson, A.,
Department of Experimental Pathology, The Medical
College of Saint Bartholomew's Hospital, Charterhouse
Square, London, UK (Ed.)

The inducible isoforms of the enzymes cyclooxygenase
(COX 2), nitric oxide synthase (iNOS) and heme oxygenase
1 (HO-1) have generated great interest as possible
therapeutic targets in inflammation. This book is the first
publication to address the importance of all three enzymes
and the consequences of their interactions to the
inflammatory process.

The book brings together overviews by leading researchers
in the field of the current status of knowledge of COX,
NOS and HO in inflammation. These overviews cover a
series of new concepts in the mechanism of inflammation.
Topics include inducible enzyme involvement in
inflammatory processes including the role in vascular
permeability, leukocyte migration, granuloma formation,
angiogenesis, neuroinflammation and algesia. New
findings from transgenic animal models are reviewed.
Other chapters address the importance of these enzymes
in inflammatory disease states including rheumatoid
arthritis, atherosclerosis and multiple sclerosis. The
possibility of selective inhibitors or inducers of COX, NOS
and HO, and their use in the clinic is discussed.

The subject matter of this book is of interest to rheumatol-
ogists, pathologists, pharmacologists, neuroscientists and
anyone with an academic interest in the mechanisms of
inflammation.

PIR – Progress in Inflammation Research
Willoughby, D. A., Tomlinson, A. (Ed.)
**Inducible Enzymes in the Inflamma-
tory Response**
1998. Approx. 200 pages. Hardcover
ISBN 3-7643-5850-5
Due in November 1998

http://www.birkhauser.ch

Check our Highlights for new and notable titles selected monthly
in each field

Contents

BioSciences with Birkhäuser

For orders originating from all over the world
except USA and Canada:

For orders originating in the USA and
Canada:

(Prices are subject to change without notice. 10/98)

Birkhäuser Verlag AG
P.O. Box 133
CH-4010 Basel / Switzerland
Fax: +41 / 61 / 205 07 92
e-mail: orders@birkhauser.ch

Birkhäuser Boston, Inc.
333 Meadowland Parkway
USA-Secaucus, NJ 07094-2491
Fax: +1 / 201 348 4033
e-mail: orders@birkhauser.com

Birkhäuser

http://www.birkhauser.ch

Check our Highlights for new and notable titles selected monthly in each field

PIR
Progress in Inflammation Research

Cytokines in Severe Sepsis and Septic Shock

Redl, H. / Schlag, G.†,
Ludwig Boltzmann Institute for Experimental and Clinical
Traumatology, Vienna, Austria

This book deals with the central role of cytokines in the generalized inflammatory response of the host as the consequence of severe infection/endotoxin action. International specialists cover several aspects in 20 chapters starting with the agents responsible (endotoxin, superantigens) and recognition during cytokine induction. Further chapters deal with the signal transduction cascade, its modulation due to sex or genetic polymorphism, and the possibilities and problems in detection (including surrogate markers). Major targets of actions are covered in the chapters on coagulation/fibrinolysis, adherence molecules, vasoactive factors, apoptosis and metabolism. As not all actions of cytokines are beneficial, several chapters deal with the prevention of induction, modulation of the cytokine generation or scavenging cytokines including gene therapy approaches. Models are necessary for obtaining pathophysiological information and for testing therapeutic approaches, and thus all chapters deal with experimental models as well as clinical trials. The reasons why these have failed so far are the subject of the final chapter.

Researchers and students of Critical Care Medicine and Biomedicine will find up-to-date reviews and data in this book.

PIR – Progress in Inflammation Research
Redl, H. / Schlag, G. †
Cytokines in Severe Sepsis and Septic Shock
1998. Approx. 300 pages. Hardcover
ISBN 3-7643-5877-7
Due in November 1998

BioSciences with Birkhäuser

(Prices are subject to change without notice. 10/98)

For orders originating from all over the world
except USA and Canada:

For orders originating in the USA and
Canada:

Birkhäuser Verlag AG
P.O. Box 133
CH-4010 Basel / Switzerland
Fax: +41 / 61 / 205 07 92
e-mail: orders@birkhauser.ch

Birkhäuser Boston, Inc.
333 Meadowland Parkway
USA-Secaucus, NJ 07094-2491
Fax: +1 / 201 348 4033
e-mail: orders@birkhauser.com

Birkhäuser

Detailed information about all our titles also available on the internet:

http://www.birkhauser.ch

Check our Highlights for new and notable titles selected monthly in each field

Methods in Pulmonary Research

Uhlig S.,
Forschungszentrum Borstel, Germany /
Taylor A.E.,
University of Southern Alabama, Mobile, AL, USA (Ed.)

Methods in Pulmonary Research presents a comprehensive review of methods used to study physiology and the cell biology of the lung. The book covers the entire range of techniques from those that require cell cultures to those using in vivo experimental models.
Up-to-date techniques such as intravital microscopy are presented. Yet standard methods such as classical short circuit techniques used to study tracheal transport are fully covered. This book will be extremely useful for all who work in pulmonary research, yet need a practical guide to incorporate other established methods into their research programs. Thus the book will prove to be a valuable resource for cell biologists who wish to use organs in their research programs as well biological scientists who are moving their research programs into more cell related phenomena.

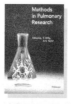

Uhlig S., Taylor A.E. (Ed.)
Methods in Pulmonary Research
1998. 544 pages. Hardcover
ISBN 3-7643-5427-5

BioSciences with Birkhäuser

(Prices are subject to change without notice. 10/98)

For orders originating from all over the world except USA and Canada:

For orders originating in the USA and Canada:

Birkhäuser Verlag AG
P.O. Box 133
CH-4010 Basel / Switzerland
Fax: +41 / 61 / 205 07 92
e-mail: orders@birkhauser.ch

Birkhäuser Boston, Inc.
333 Meadowland Parkway
USA-Secaucus, NJ 07094-2491
Fax: +1 / 201 348 4033
e-mail: orders@birkhauser.com

Birkhäuser